CONCISE GUIDE TO

Child and Adolescent Psychiatry

Fourth Edition

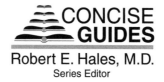

CONCISE GUIDES

Robert E. Hales, M.D.

Series Editor

CONCISE GUIDE TO

Child and Adolescent Psychiatry

Fourth Edition

Mina K. Dulcan, M.D.

MaryBeth Lake, M.D.

American
Psychiatric
Publishing, Inc.

Washington, DC
London, England

Note: The authors have worked to ensure that all information in this book is accurate at the time of publication and consistent with general psychiatric and medical standards, and that information concerning drug dosages, schedules, and routes of administration is accurate at the time of publication and consistent with standards set by the U.S. Food and Drug Administration and the general medical community. As medical research and practice continue to advance, however, therapeutic standards may change. Moreover, specific situations may require a specific therapeutic response not included in this book. For these reasons and because human and mechanical errors sometimes occur, we recommend that readers follow the advice of physicians directly involved in their care or the care of a member of their family.

Books published by American Psychiatric Publishing, Inc., represent the views and opinions of the individual authors and do not necessarily represent the policies and opinions of APPI or the American Psychiatric Association.

Diagnostic criteria included in this book are reprinted, with permission, from *Diagnostic and Statistical Manual of Mental Disorders,* 4th Edition, Text Revision. Copyright © 2000, American Psychiatric Association.

Manufactured in the United States of America on acid-free paper
15   14   13   12   11   5   4   3   2   1
Fourth Edition

American Psychiatric Publishing, Inc.
1000 Wilson Boulevard
Arlington, VA 22209-3901
www.appi.org

Typeset in Adobe's Times and Helvetica

Library of Congress Cataloging-in-Publication Data
Dulcan, Mina K.
　Concise guide to child and adolescent psychiatry / Mina K. Dulcan, MaryBeth Lake. — 4th ed.
　　p. ; cm. — (Concise guides series)
　　Child and adolescent psychiatry
　　Includes bibliographical references and index.
　　ISBN 978-1-58562-416-4 (pbk. : alk. paper) 1. Child psychiatry—Handbooks, manuals, etc. 2. Adolescent psychiatry—Handbooks, manuals, etc. I. Lake, MaryBeth, 1966– II. Title. III. Title: Child and adolescent psychiatry. IV. Series: Concise guides (American Psychiatric Publishing)
　　[DNLM: 1. Adolescent Psychiatry—methods—Handbooks. 2. Child Psychiatry—methods—Handbooks. 3. Adolescent. 4. Child. 5. Mental Disorders—Handbooks. WS 39]
　　RJ499.3.D84 2012
　　618.92'89--dc23

2011015820

British Library Cataloguing in Publication Data
A CIP record is available from the British Library.

CONTENTS

3 Axis I Disorders Usually First Diagnosed in Infancy, Childhood, or Adolescence: Attention-Deficit and Disruptive Behavior Disorders

5 "Adult" Disorders That May Begin in Childhood or Adolescence 99

9 Psychosocial Treatments 313

LIST OF TABLES

4   Other Axis I Disorders Usually First Diagnosed in Infancy, Childhood, or Adolescence

5   "Adult" Disorders That May Begin in Childhood or Adolescence

ABOUT THE AUTHORS

Mina K. Dulcan, M.D.

Margaret C. Osterman Professor of Child Psychiatry; Head, Department of Child and Adolescent Psychiatry, Children's Memorial Hospital; Director, Warren Wright Adolescent Program, Northwestern Memorial Hospital; Professor of Psychiatry and Behavioral Sciences and Pediatrics; Chief, Child and Adolescent Psychiatry, Northwestern University, Feinberg School of Medicine, Chicago, Illinois

MaryBeth Lake, M.D.

Director of Education in Child and Adolescent Psychiatry, Department of Child and Adolescent Psychiatry, Children's Memorial Hospital; Associate Professor of Psychiatry and Behavioral Sciences, Northwestern University, Feinberg School of Medicine, Chicago, Illinois

INTRODUCTION

to the Concise Guides Series

The Concise Guides Series from American Psychiatric Publishing, Inc., provides, in an accessible format, practical information for psychiatrists, psychiatry residents, and medical students working in a variety of treatment settings, such as inpatient psychiatry units, outpatient clinics, consultation-liaison services, and private office settings. The Concise Guides are meant to complement the more detailed information to be found in lengthier psychiatry texts.

The Concise Guides address topics of special concern to psychiatrists in clinical practice. The books in this series contain a detailed table of contents, along with an index, tables, figures, and other charts for easy access. The books are designed to fit into a lab coat pocket or jacket pocket, which makes them a convenient source of information. References have been limited to those most relevant to the material presented.

Robert E. Hales, M.D., M.B.A.
Series Editor, Concise Guides

PREFACE TO THE FOURTH EDITION

Time flies! Since the publication in 2003 of the third edition of the *Concise Guide to Child and Adolescent Psychiatry,* the field of child mental health has moved at an ever-accelerating pace. The body of clinical research and empirically supported treatments has grown, evaluation practices have been refined, awareness of emotional and behavioral problems in youth has increased, progress has been made in decreasing the stigma of mental illness and obtaining parity for insurance coverage, and the lay media have been flooded with controversies regarding psychiatric disorders and their treatments.

Findings that most experts agree are relevant to clinical practice have been distilled and incorporated into this new edition, and other material has been pruned. Each section of the book has been revised and updated. The American Psychiatric Association has graciously permitted the reprinting of tables of diagnostic criteria from DSM-IV-TR.

■ ACKNOWLEDGMENTS

Rich Martini, who made important contributions to the second and third editions, has moved on to Salt Lake City, where he is leading the child and adolescent psychiatry program at Primary Children's Medical Center. We are deeply grateful to all of the child and adolescent psychiatry fellows and the faculty and staff in the Department of Child and Adolescent Psychiatry at Children's Memorial Hospital, who inspire us to learn more and who teach us every day.

INTRODUCTION

The *Concise Guide to Child and Adolescent Psychiatry,* Fourth Edition, offers an introduction to mental health care in children and adolescents to be used in conjunction with clinical supervision and consultation. This book was written to be used as a primer on child and adolescent psychiatry for medical and other health or mental health students or clinical trainees and as a brief update for practicing physicians, nurses, and advanced practice nurses in general psychiatry, child and adolescent psychiatry, pediatrics, neurology, and family medicine. It may also be useful for professionals in special education, child welfare, and juvenile justice, as well as parents. In the interest of brevity, complex theoretical notions, new research, and areas of controversy have been simplified. Each section on a disorder or clinical situation includes a listing of relevant treatment methods. Treatment techniques are described in Chapters 8 and 9. Each chapter has additional reading for those who wish more detail. For more in-depth, comprehensive coverage of child mental health, see *Dulcan's Textbook of Child and Adolescent Psychiatry* (Dulcan 2010). The American Academy of Child and Adolescent Psychiatry practice parameters—clinical guidelines that are based upon the scientific literature and the wisdom of experienced clinicians—are published in the *Journal of the American Academy of Child and Adolescent Psychiatry.* They are cited in the corresponding chapters.

Throughout this book, *children* refers to both prepubertal children and adolescents, unless otherwise specified. *Parent* is used for the child's primary adult caregiver(s), whoever that may be.

■ CHANGE IN CHILDREN AND ADOLESCENTS

The primary "work" of children is to grow and change in multiple dimensions. Rigid descriptions of mental disorders and psychiatric symptoms do not capture the liveliness and energy of children as they develop and cope with internal and external difficulties. A child's tendency to change is a therapeutic ally. As clinicians, we work with the natural dynamics of the interaction between our interventions and developmental processes.

All disorders in childhood can exert lasting effects beyond the boundaries of the primary psychiatric disorder. Developmental complications are often cumulative and may disrupt a wide range of functions. Social, cognitive, and psychological development, and even physical growth (Pine et al. 1996) may be impaired. Progressive learning delays, school failure, low self-esteem, demoralization, impaired relationships with family members, and rejection or neglect by peers are common complications of childhood-onset disorders. Prompt intervention can reduce these developmental consequences.

Regardless of the etiology of the primary disorder, biological, cognitive, psychodynamic, familial, social, economic, and cultural factors are critical in determining the course of illness. Genes can interact with environment to increase vulnerability or to reduce risk. The effects of early developmental deficits may be compensated for or exacerbated by later opportunities or barriers. The family or social environment can amplify strengths or aggravate weaknesses. The adult outcome of a childhood disorder in a specific patient is a result of the interaction among therapeutic forces and risk and protective factors. The ultimate prognosis may depend more on the ability of the child and family to learn to cope with the illness than on the severity of the disorder. Resilient individuals may even turn childhood symptoms such as excessive sensitivity (separation anxiety disorder), unrelenting stubbornness (oppositional defiant disorder), or uncontrolled activity and enthusiasm (attention-deficit/hyperactivity disorder) into strengths in adulthood. Compensatory abilities and an enhancing environment can result in achievement and adaptation far above that predicted from early deficits.

■ OVERVIEW OF DIAGNOSIS

Use of DSM-IV-TR for Children and Adolescents

"Adult" psychiatric disorders in DSM-IV-TR (American Psychiatric Association 2000) can begin during childhood. Any Axis I diagnosis can be used for a child if the criteria are met. Some disorders have slightly adapted criteria for children. The DSM-IV-TR "disorders usually first diagnosed in infancy, childhood, or adolescence" include diagnoses that typically begin in childhood. Some behavior patterns are normal at certain developmental stages but become pathological if they persist (becoming, for example, separation anxiety disorder, functional enuresis, functional encopresis, or oppositional defiant disorder). Most Axis I disorders, however, are not "normal" at any age. The only Axis II disorder in the childhood section of DSM-IV-TR is mental retardation. Pervasive developmental disorders (including autistic disorder) and specific developmental disorders (learning, motor skills, and communication disorders) are on Axis I. In this book, key DSM-IV-TR criteria for each disorder are highlighted. For full details, refer to DSM-IV-TR (American Psychiatric Association 2000).

DSM-IV-TR contains a variety of clinical circumstances, classified as "V codes" or "other conditions that may be a focus of clinical attention," that are not psychiatric diagnoses but may prompt assessment and treatment. Any of these codes may be used for children's conditions, but some are especially common in clinical settings. The most prevalent conditions are listed in Table 1–1, and many are discussed in Chapter 7, "Special Clinical Circumstances." Although some clinicians are tempted to use V codes to avoid "labeling" a child, these categories should be used only if the child's symptoms do not meet the criteria for another DSM-IV-TR disorder.

All DSM-IV-TR diagnoses (except for tic disorders) require evidence that the symptoms are causing significant distress or impairment in social, academic, or occupational functioning.

Medical conditions are listed on Axis III. The full range of medical problems, from a fever or earache to a brain tumor, may be

TABLE 1–1.	**DSM-IV-TR conditions especially relevant to children and adolescents that may be a focus of clinical attention**

Relational problem related to a mental disorder or general medical condition
Parent–child relational problem
Sibling relational problem

Physical abuse of child
Sexual abuse of child
Neglect of child

Noncompliance with treatment
Child or adolescent antisocial behavior
Borderline intellectual functioning (coded on Axis II) (IQ 71–84)
Bereavement
Academic problem
Identity problem

Source. American Psychiatric Association 2000.

signaled first by behavioral or emotional symptoms or declining school performance. Children with chronic medical disorders or physical disabilities are at increased risk for psychiatric disorders (see Chapter 7).

Axis IV is used for reporting psychosocial and environmental problems relevant to diagnosis, treatment, and prognosis. Stressors with unique effects during development include parental absence or neglect, physical and sexual abuse, psychiatric disorder in a caregiver, and puberty. On Axis V, the clinician uses the Global Assessment of Functioning Scale (GAF) to rate the lowest level of functioning for the past week. The Children's Global Assessment Scale (Shaffer et al. 1983) may be used to supplement the GAF.

Comorbidity

Psychiatric disorders typically occur in combinations. This is true not only in young people treated in the most intensive settings, such as inpatient units and residential treatment facilities, but also in outpatients. Comorbidity is common even in community epidemiological surveys, although less so than in children who have been referred for clinical services. Combinations of disorders may be unexpected, such as a youth with impulsive hyperactivity or aggressive conduct problems who also suffers from depression or anxiety. Broad-spectrum rating scales are a useful supplement to the diagnostic process, to avoid overly narrow focus on the presenting problem.

■ OVERVIEW OF TREATMENT

Until recently, psychiatric treatment in children was more an art than a science. Treatment methods were applied regardless of diagnosis and reflected the training and beliefs of the therapist rather than the characteristics of the patient. Newer trends include consideration of biological factors, multimodal treatment approaches, multidisciplinary teams, and use of evidence-based interventions. With improvements in diagnostic criteria and evaluation techniques and the design and rigorous testing of therapy models and medications for specific disorders, treatment selection is increasingly scientific.

In contrast to treatment in adults, a child is typically brought to the clinical setting by someone else. Although the child is identified as "the patient," each case has at least two clients: a parent or guardian and the child, whose needs and desires may conflict. In addition, treatment often involves other family members; teachers and school counselors; government agencies, such as child protective services or the juvenile court; community organizations; and financial providers, such as welfare, Medicaid, and insurance companies. Because children depend on adults for their basic needs and have little autonomy in choosing caregivers, residence, schools, or activities, the clinician must work in partnership with the parents and other support systems to reestablish developmental progress and maximize adaptive outcome.

■ REFERENCES

American Psychiatric Association: Diagnostic and Statistical Manual of Mental Disorders, 4th Edition, Text Revision. Washington, DC, American Psychiatric Association, 2000

Dulcan MK (ed): Dulcan's Textbook of Child and Adolescent Psychiatry. Washington, DC, American Psychiatric Publishing, 2010

Pine DS, Cohen P, Brook J: Emotional problems during youth as predictors of stature during early adulthood: results from a prospective epidemiologic study. Pediatrics 97:856–863, 1996

Shaffer D, Gould MS, Brasic J, et al: A Children's Global Assessment Scale (CGAS). Arch Gen Psychiatry 40:1228–1231, 1983

■ ADDITIONAL READING

Rapoport JL, Ismond DR: DSM-IV Training Guide for Diagnosis of Childhood Disorders. New York, Brunner/Mazel, 1996

EVALUATION AND TREATMENT PLANNING

■ EVALUATION

A comprehensive evaluation includes obtaining a biopsychosocial history (see Table 2–1); performing a mental status examination; ordering any additional tests; and obtaining records (with parental permission) from the child's school, pediatrician, and agencies such as child protective services or the juvenile court. The clinician should request reports of all prior psychiatric, psychological, developmental, and medical evaluations and treatment. Assessment should continue throughout the course of treatment as the child, parents, and situation change. When the presenting problems are urgent or narrowly circumscribed, treatment may be initiated after a focused evaluation with more complete assessment as time permits.

Before the evaluation, the clinician should tell the parents how long the evaluation will take, what it will cost, and what they can expect at the end. The clinician should advise parents on how to prepare the child for the first visit. Some parents invite the child out for an ice-cream cone but bring him or her to the child psychiatry clinic instead. Needless to say, this does not enhance the child's cooperation, although it does provide the clinician with useful data about the parents.

In conducting an evaluation, the clinician must constantly be mindful of the patient's developmental level, which determines whether a behavior (e.g., temper tantrums, separation anxiety) is pathological. Developmental stage influences the nature of symp-

TABLE 2–1.   **Outline of biopsychosocial history**

Chief symptom and reasons for referral

History of present illness

Development of the symptoms

Attitudes of child and parents toward the symptoms

Effects of the symptoms on the child and family

Stressors

Prior psychological or psychiatric evaluations

Prior treatment

Psychotherapy: type, frequency, duration, effects

Medication: exact doses, schedule, beneficial and adverse effects

Intensive treatments such as hospitalization or residential placement

Environmental changes and effects

Current developmental status

Motor abilities and activity level

Attention

Speech and language

Academic performance

Relationships with peers

Risk-taking behaviors

Sexual development and behavior

Hobbies, activities, athletic interests and skills

Relationships with family members and other significant adults

Review of behavioral and psychological symptoms

Medical review of systems

Past history

Psychiatric

Medical

Neurological

Developmental history

Pregnancy and delivery

Neonatal period, infancy, early childhood

Temperament

Milestones

Motor

Cognitive

Speech and language

Social

TABLE 2–1.	Outline of biopsychosocial history *(continued)*

Developmental history *(continued)*
    School history
    Traumatic events
Psychosocial and psychiatric history of each parent
Developmental history of the couple/family life cycle stage
Family medical history
Current family circumstances, concerns, liabilities, resources

toms, expectable reactions to stressors, ability to communicate and to understand concepts, and capacity to participate in different types of treatment.

The structure of an evaluation is determined by the child's age, the nature of the presenting problems, and practical factors. It is often useful to begin by meeting briefly with the child and parents together, to clarify and understand each person's views of the presenting problems and the goals of the evaluation and to develop an initial impression of family interaction. For children younger than 6 years, it may be convenient to obtain the entire history from the parents before seeing the child. Older children, especially adolescents, should be involved early in the evaluation process. Adolescents are often concerned about confidentiality and should be told that what they say will be shared only with their permission, unless they are at risk for physical harm, such as from suicide, homicide, substance abuse, high-risk sexual behavior, or running away. Clinicians are legally mandated to report suspected physical or sexual abuse to child protection authorities.

Use of Multiple Informants

No single informant or technique can give a full description of a child. Children, teachers, parents, other relatives, community members, and clinicians each have their own point of view and opportunities for observation. Lack of agreement between parents and teachers or between two parents often results from genuine variations in the behavior of children in different settings and with different people. Ideally, both parents should be interviewed, even if they are not living together, because their cooperation will enhance the likelihood of successful treatment, and each parent has a unique perspective on the child's development and environment. A telephone interview may be substituted if a parent is not available in person.

History From Parents

The elements of a complete history from the parents or caregivers are outlined in Table 2–1. The construction of a time line, including symptoms, life events, and changes in the family and environment, can help organize a complex history.

An important element in the developmental history is the child's *temperament,* or "style" of behavior. Children can be rated on each of the nine dimensions listed in Table 2–2. The *goodness of fit* between the child's temperament and the parents' temperament, expectations, and child-rearing skills significantly affects developmental course and outcome. In addition, certain trait clusters (Table 2–3) have predictive value. Both *difficult* and *slow-to-warm-up* children are at risk for emotional and behavior problems, whereas *easy* children are relatively protected.

TABLE 2–2.   **Dimensions of temperament**

---

1. Activity level
2. Rhythmicity (regularity and predictability of biological functions)
3. Approach to or withdrawal from novel stimuli
4. Adaptability to environmental change
5. Intensity of reaction
6. Threshold of responsiveness (intensity of stimulation required to evoke a response)
7. Quality of mood (positive, neutral, or negative)
8. Distractibility
9. Attention span and persistence

Source.   Adapted from Thomas A, Chess S: *Temperament in Clinical Practice.* New York, Guilford, 1986.

TABLE 2–3.	**Temperament clusters**

Easy

    Positive mood

    Regular biological rhythms

    Adaptable

    Low intensity of reactions

    Positive approach to novelty

Difficult

    Negative mood

    Irregular biological rhythms

    Slow to adapt

    Intense reactions

    Negative response to novelty

Slow to warm up

    Gradual adaptation after repeated contact

    Mild intensity of reactions

    Negative response to novelty

Source.   Adapted from Thomas A, Chess S: *Temperament in Clinical Practice.* New York, Guilford, 1986.

Patient Interview

During the patient interview, the child provides his or her view of the history and current symptoms, strengths, and concerns and the clinician makes observations. Children and adolescents often report their anxiety and depression, clandestine conduct problems, and drug use more accurately than their parents do. Parents typically report history, observable behavior problems, and family background more accurately than the child does. The details of the interview vary with developmental stage. The content of the mental status examination is outlined in Table 2–4.

The therapist should begin the patient interview by informally discussing nonthreatening topics before focusing on the presenting symptoms. For patients who are not very verbal, an opportunity to draw (with pencils, crayons, or washable markers) can help them feel comfortable enough to engage in conversation. Young children ini-

TABLE 2–4.   **Mental status examination**

Physical appearance and grooming
Interactions with clinician
Understanding of the purpose of the interview
Motor activity level and coordination
Tics, stereotypies, mannerisms
Mood and affect
Anxiety
Obsessions or compulsions
Attention, persistence, frustration tolerance
Impulsivity
Oppositionality
Verbal or physical aggression
Speech and language
Hallucinations, delusions, thought disorder
Clinical estimate of intelligence
Judgment and insight

tially may want the parent to be present and may be more comfortable with play materials (e.g., dollhouse, stuffed animals, blocks, clay) than with a formal interview. Some clinicians previously believed that asking children direct questions about their symptoms was harmful, but research has disproved this theory. Clinicians must ask children direct questions (using wording that is adapted to the child's developmental level) to understand their emotional states.

Family Evaluation

Each person living with the patient, as well as noncustodial parents, grandparents, and siblings who are no longer living at home, may be crucial to understanding family dynamics, including both unexpected sources of emotional support and areas of conflict. Meeting simultaneously with all significant family members to collect information and to observe interactions is often useful. Families with young children may benefit from the use of role playing, family drawings, or puppet play. The clinician may ask the family to complete a

TABLE 2–5.	**Family developmental tasks**

Forming a "marital coalition" to meet the needs of the adults for intimacy, sexuality, and emotional support

Establishing a "parental coalition" to form flexible relationships with children and present a consistent disciplinary front

Emphasizing nurturance, enculturation, and emancipation of children

Coping with crises

Source. Adapted from Fleck S: "A General Systems Approach to Severe Family Pathology." *American Journal of Psychiatry* 133:669–673, 1973.

task during the session in order to assess family interactions. A family tree or genogram helps the clinician to organize data on family members and their relationships.

Regardless of a family's structure or members, the well-being of the child requires that certain tasks be accomplished (Table 2–5). Well-functioning families respond resiliently to stress, communicate effectively, assign roles that suit the needs and abilities of each family member, respond appropriately to emotions, solve problems both within and outside the boundaries of the family, and find effective and humane ways to control the behavior of family members.

Tasks of the initial session of a family assessment include the following:

• Ascertain family members' views of the problem.
• Begin to establish a relationship with each family member to facilitate the treatment alliance.
• Gather data by observation and with questions.
• Make test interventions and assess their effects.
• Propose and negotiate a provisional plan for the next steps.

Mental health care for young people is unlikely to succeed without considering their parents' needs. Parents struggling with their own untreated psychiatric disorders may be unable to meet the child's emotional and physical needs, and there may be a "contagious" effect on the child. The clinician's most important contribution may be to arrange for the parent to receive psychiatric assessment and pharmacological and/or psychotherapeutic treatment. The clinician may need to use both empathy and judicious persuasion to induce the parent to assume a "patient" role.

Standardized Evaluation Instruments

Selected parent, teacher, and self-report behavior checklists, questionnaires, and rating scales supplement the clinical evaluation by providing a systematic review of behaviors and psychiatric symptoms. Scores may be compared with norms obtained from large community-based samples or groups of clinically referred children. Ratings may also be done at intervals to measure progress. The most commonly used broad-spectrum package consists of the Child Behavior Checklist (CBCL) parent rating form, the Teacher Report Form (TRF), and the Youth Self-Report (YSR) Form (Achenbach System of Empirically Based Assessment; http://www.aseba.org). More specific instruments are available for one or more diagnoses. Structured and semistructured diagnostic interview protocols (see Table 2–6) are more commonly used in research but often have clinical usefulness.

TABLE 2–6.   **Examples of standardized diagnostic assessment interviews**

Structured diagnostic interview
   Diagnostic Interview Schedule for Children (DISC)
Semistructured diagnostic interviews
   Diagnostic Interview for Children and Adolescents (DICA)
   Schedule for Affective Disorders and Schizophrenia for School-Aged
      Children and Adolescents (Kiddie-SADS)

Note.   For references and more detail, see *Journal of the American Academy of Child and Adolescent Psychiatry,* Special Section: Diagnostic Interviews, 39:1, January 2000.

Medical Evaluation

A standard evaluation includes a medical history and physical examination (within the past year or more recently if the onset of problems is acute) to identify any medical causes of symptoms or coexisting medical disorders. Neurological consultation or testing (e.g., electroencephalogram, brain scan) is indicated only if focal neurological signs or symptoms are present or if the history suggests seizures, regression in cognitive or physical functioning, or sequelae of brain injury. Laboratory tests may be obtained, especially if pharmacological treatment is anticipated. Urine testing for drugs and, in female adolescents, a pregnancy test are often indicated. Scientific evidence does not support the use of brain imaging in clinical diagnosis or treatment of psychiatric disorders in youth.

School Assessment

School reports are almost always useful. Attention, learning, quality and quantity of homework and classwork, behavior in class and on the playground, and social relationships are sensitive indicators of the presence of psychiatric symptoms and of developmental status. After obtaining parental consent, the clinician may talk with the teacher or school counselor, obtain school records (educational testing, behavior, grades, and attendance), arrange for teachers to complete standardized checklists, and perhaps even visit the school to observe the youngster.

Psychological Testing

Standardized tests administered by a clinical psychologist can assess intellectual potential, cognitive skills, and fund of knowledge (Table 2–7). Individually administered tests provide a more accurate evaluation than those given to children in the classroom. Tests have been criticized because of cultural influences on performance, unresponsiveness to "creative" responses, the dangers of using a rigid construct of intelligence that masks individual strengths, the use of test results to exclude children from mainstream education, and potential insults to developing self-esteem. Despite these concerns, IQ

TABLE 2–7. Individually administered tests of intellectual capacity, learning, and adaptive functioning

Intelligence

Differential Ability Scales, Second Edition (DAS-II)	2.6–17 years Subtests estimate General Cognitive Ability (GCA) and the subdomains of Verbal, Nonverbal, and Spatial Ability
Kaufman Adolescent and Adult Intelligence Test (KAIT)	11 years through adulthood Distinguishes between learned information and capacity to solve novel problems
Kaufman Assessment Battery for Children, Second Edition (K-ABC-II)	3–18 years Subtests estimate general Mental Processing and the subdomains of Sequential and Simultaneous Processing, Learning, Planning, and Knowledge
Kaufman Brief Intelligence Test (K-BIT)	Screening test to estimate IQ
Leiter International Performance Scale—Revised	2–20 years Nonverbal test for use with persons who are hearing impaired or autistic or who do not speak English
Peabody Picture Vocabulary Test, Fourth Edition (PPVT-4)	2.6 years through adulthood Brief test of receptive vocabulary used to estimate verbal intelligence
Shipley-2	7 years through adulthood Brief pencil-and-paper test that does not require a psychologist to administer Subtests estimate general cognitive functioning and the subdomains of Crystallized/Verbal and Fluid/Nonverbal cognitive ability

TABLE 2–7. **Individually administered tests of intellectual capacity, learning, and adaptive functioning** *(continued)*

Stanford-Binet Intelligence Scale, Fifth Edition	2 years through adulthood Subtests estimate Verbal IQ, Nonverbal IQ, and Full Scale IQ, as well as the subdomains of Fluid Reasoning, Knowledge, Quantitative Reasoning, Visual Spatial Processing, and Working Memory
Universal Nonverbal Intelligence Test (UNIT)	5–17 years Subtests estimate Full Scale IQ and the subdomains of Memory, Reasoning, Symbolic, and Non-Symbolic Ability
Wechsler Abbreviated Scale of Intelligence (WASI)	6 years through adulthood Both 4-subtest and 2-subtest versions estimate Full Scale IQ; 4-subtest version also estimates Verbal and Performance IQ
Wechsler Adult Intelligence Scale, Fourth Edition (WAIS-IV)	16 years through adulthood Subtests estimate Full Scale IQ and the subdomains of Verbal Comprehension, Perceptual Reasoning, Working Memory, and Processing Speed
Wechsler Intelligence Scale for Children, Fourth Edition (WISC-IV)	6–16 years Subtests estimate Full Scale IQ and the subdomains of Verbal Comprehension, Perceptual Reasoning, Working Memory, and Processing Speed
Wechsler Preschool and Primary Scale of Intelligence, Third Edition (WPPSI-III)	2.6–7.3 years Subtests are grouped into verbal and performance scales

TABLE 2–7. Individually administered tests of intellectual capacity, learning, and adaptive functioning *(continued)*

Intelligence *(continued)*

Woodcock-Johnson Tests of Cognitive Ability—Third Revision	2 years through adulthood
	Frequently used by schools
	Subtests estimate General Intellectual Ability and the subdomains of Verbal Ability, Thinking Ability, and Cognitive Efficiency

Academic achievement

Kaufman Test of Educational Achievement, Second Edition (K-TEA-II)	4.6 years through adulthood
	Subtests estimate academic mastery of reading, writing, math, and oral language skills
Wechsler Individual Achievement Tests, Second Edition (WIAT-II)	5–19 years
	Brief (screener) version estimates skills in reading, math reasoning, and spelling
	Comprehensive Battery adds listening comprehension and written and oral expression
Wide Range Achievement Test, Fourth Edition (WRAT-4)	5 years through adulthood
	Subtests screen for academic mastery of reading, writing, math, and oral comprehension skills
Woodcock-Johnson III Tests of Achievement	2 years through adulthood
	Subtests estimate academic mastery of reading, writing, math, academic knowledge, and oral language skills

TABLE 2–7. Individually administered tests of intellectual capacity, learning, and adaptive functioning *(continued)*

Adaptive behavior (required to diagnose mental retardation)

Adaptive Behavior Assessment System, Second Edition (ABAS-II)

Birth through adulthood

Estimates overall adaptive functioning (General Adaptive Composite) and functioning in the subdomains of Conceptual, Social, and Practical skills

Parent and teacher report forms

Vineland Adaptive Behavior Scales, Second Edition

Birth through adulthood

Semistructured interview with parent (or brief written form for teacher)

Estimates overall adaptive functioning (Adaptive Behavior Composite) and functioning in the subdomains of Communication, Daily Living Skills, Socialization, and Motor Skills

Woodcock-Johnson Scales of Independent Behavior—Revised (SIB-R)

Birth through adulthood

Semistructured interview with caregiver

Estimates overall adaptive functioning (Broad Independence Index) and functioning in the subdomains of Motor, Social Interaction and Communication, Personal Living, and Community Living skills tests provide a global assessment that has clinical predictive value, particularly when combined with an evaluation of adaptive behavior. Projective tests such as the Children's Apperception Test (CAT) or the Rorschach Inkblot Technique are not useful in making diagnostic or treatment decisions. The most commonly used test for assessing infants (ages birth to 3 years) is the Bayley Scales of Infant Development, Third Edition. It is used to evaluate motor (fine and gross), language (receptive and expressive), and cognitive development.

Neuropsychological testing uses a neurodiagnostic battery of tests to provide a detailed assessment of a patient's cognitive strengths and weaknesses and compare them with patterns seen in individuals with developmental, neurological, or other medical conditions. It can assist in the diagnosis, localization, and monitoring of neurodevelopmental, neurodegenerative, or acquired disorders of brain functioning or adverse effects of treatments such as cranial radiation and chemotherapy. Neuropsychological testing is not indicated as a diagnostic procedure for attention-deficit/hyperactivity disorder, although it can assist in the assessment of specific learning disabilities.

■ TREATMENT PLANNING

Treatment plans are based on both psychiatric diagnosis and identified target symptoms. The strengths and vulnerabilities of the patient and the resources and liabilities of the family are critical factors in treatment planning. The social environment, including school, neighborhood, and social support networks, strongly influences choice of treatment strategy. The practical realities of the quality and availability of community resources and the family's ability to pay for or to attend treatment sessions often compel the clinician to modify an "ideal" or comprehensive plan. Realistic and efficient selection and sequencing of treatment modalities are central to effective decision making. Clinical judgments regarding anticipated treatment effectiveness, efficiency, and risk–benefit ratio may lead to selection of a single form of treatment or multimodal therapies. Interventions may be administered simultaneously or sequentially, as the child or family requires or is able to make use of additional treatment.

Parental motivation or ability to carry out the treatment plan may strongly influence treatment decisions. For example, unusual strengths of a family may avert hospitalization of a psychotic or suicidal child or limitations may prevent implementation of family therapy or maintenance of the child living at home. For children from disrupted homes or abusive or neglectful environments, the first priority may not be psychiatric care, but social services, such as a safe and stable home, food, supervision, and medical care. In complex cases, a case manager who coordinates the involvement of various agencies and services (sometimes called "wraparound") may be able to maintain a child in the community, which may result in a better outcome at a lower overall cost.

Each of a child's symptoms may appear to call for a different intervention. In setting priorities, factors to consider include the following:

- Risk of physical harm to the child or to others
- Symptoms that will likely increase in severity and chronicity if not treated rapidly (e.g., school avoidance)
- Patient and family motivation and resistance
- Symptoms or family members that are most accessible to treatment
- Problems that are most urgent to the patient or family

Treatment planning is an ongoing process. Continual reassessment is necessary as the effects of interventions are seen and as additional information about the child and family comes to light.

■ FEEDBACK

The clinician's findings and recommendations are typically presented to both the parents and the child. The clinician decides whether to meet with them together or separately, and in what order. Depending on the ability of each to listen or understand, parents and child are educated about the nature of the child's and the family's strengths, psychiatric liabilities or disorders, and the expected course and possible complications of the disorder. The clinician should answer questions about etiology at the level that scientific knowledge allows, while assiduously avoiding blaming or being judgmental. Parents and many children already feel guilty about real or perceived failures, and the empathic clinician is cautious to ameliorate these feelings.

Parents, and usually the child, should help determine which treatment strategy to follow. The clinician describes recommended and alternative interventions in terms of the process (duration, costs) and the anticipated benefits and risks. A successful feedback conference helps the family to understand their strengths and weaknesses, respect their child's abilities and the difficulties he or she faces, sense the interplay of multiple etiological factors, realize the implications of the child's diagnosis and prognosis, ponder the practicalities involved, acknowledge hopes and fears, and integrate the recommendations with the rest of their lives. Even the best treatment has little chance of success without the cooperation of the family and the child (to the extent possible for developmental stage and psychopathology). The treatment plan should be consistent with the family's resources. Finding areas in which improvement may be quickly attained builds the family's confidence in themselves and in the therapeutic process.

■ ADDITIONAL READING

American Academy of Child and Adolescent Psychiatry: Practice parameters for the psychiatric assessment of infants and toddlers (0–36 months). J Am Acad Child Adolesc Psychiatry 36 (suppl):21S–36S, 1997

Cepeda C: Concise Guide to the Psychiatric Interview of Children and Adolescents. Washington, DC, American Psychiatric Press, 2000

Dulcan MK (ed): Dulcan's Textbook of Child and Adolescent Psychiatry. Washington, DC, American Psychiatric Publishing, 2010

Gerson R, McGoldrick M, Petry S: Genograms: Assessment and Intervention, 3rd Edition. New York, WW Norton, 2008

3

AXIS I DISORDERS USUALLY FIRST DIAGNOSED IN INFANCY, CHILDHOOD, OR ADOLESCENCE

Attention-Deficit and Disruptive Behavior Disorders

DSM-IV-TR (American Psychiatric Association 2000) has a separate section for those disorders that typically begin before adulthood. Mental retardation (coded on Axis II) and the learning, motor skills, and communication disorders (Axis I) are presumed to be present at birth and to become symptomatic as expectations for competence increase with age. They are covered in Chapter 6, along with the pervasive developmental disorders. Reactive attachment disorder, rumination disorder, and pica characteristically begin during infancy. Attention-deficit/hyperactivity disorder (ADHD) and oppositional defiant disorder (ODD) most often appear in early childhood, whereas conduct disorder (CD) and tic disorders develop in middle childhood through adolescence. Enuresis and encopresis are diagnosed in early childhood when developmentally appropriate stages of toilet training are not achieved. Separation anxiety disorder and selective mutism become apparent when age-appropriate independent social behavior is impaired. This chapter covers attention-deficit and disruptive behavior disorders. The remaining diagnoses in this section of DSM-IV-TR are covered in Chapter 4.

In DSM-IV-TR, disruptive behavior disorder includes CD and ODD. Unlike ADHD, these disorders are characterized by willful disobedience. CD and ODD often present concurrently with ADHD, however. All three of these conditions are sometimes called *externalizing disorders,* emphasizing the prominence of externally directed behaviors. Parents and teachers are generally more distressed than the child, who often denies symptoms, blames others for problems, and is reluctant to undergo treatment. These syndromes are characterized by the chronicity and severity of clusters of problem behaviors that differentiate them from the mild behavior problems often seen in typical children.

■ ATTENTION-DEFICIT/HYPERACTIVITY DISORDER

Clinical Description

The syndrome of hyperactivity, impulsivity, and inattention was historically labeled "minimal brain damage," "minimal brain dysfunction," "hyperkinetic syndrome," "hyperactivity," or "ADD."

DSM-IV-TR defines three subtypes of ADHD: combined type (meeting criteria for both inattention and hyperactivity–impulsivity), predominantly inattentive type, and predominantly hyperactive–impulsive type (Table 3–1). The predominantly inattentive type is similar, but not identical, to the DSM-III (American Psychiatric Association 1980) category of attention-deficit disorder without hyperactivity. Children with the predominantly inattentive subtype tend to be described as "daydreamers" or "spacey," more often have comorbid anxiety and depression, are more likely to be neglected by peers, have fewer conduct and behavior problems, and present less frequently to psychiatric settings than do those with the combined type. The predominantly hyperactive–impulsive group consists largely of very young children for whom the inattention criteria are not yet developmentally appropriate. The prior diagnostic term, "attention-deficit disorder" (ADD), is no longer correct but is used in the lay media, sometimes to refer to inattentive-type ADHD, and sometimes for the entire syndrome.

TABLE 3–1.   **DSM-IV-TR diagnostic criteria for attention-deficit/hyperactivity disorder**

A. Either (1) or (2):

(1) six (or more) of the following symptoms of **inattention** have persisted for at least 6 months to a degree that is maladaptive and inconsistent with developmental level:

Inattention

(a) often fails to give close attention to details or makes careless mistakes in schoolwork, work, or other activities

(b) often has difficulty sustaining attention in tasks or play activities

(c) often does not seem to listen when spoken to directly

(d) often does not follow through on instructions and fails to finish schoolwork, chores, or duties in the workplace (not due to oppositional behavior or failure to understand instructions)

(e) often has difficulty organizing tasks and activities

(f) often avoids, dislikes, or is reluctant to engage in tasks that require sustained mental effort (such as schoolwork or homework)

(g) often loses things necessary for tasks or activities (e.g., toys, school assignments, pencils, books, or tools)

(h) is often easily distracted by extraneous stimuli

(i) is often forgetful in daily activities

(2) six (or more) of the following symptoms of **hyperactivity–impulsivity** have persisted for at least 6 months to a degree that is maladaptive and inconsistent with developmental level:

Hyperactivity

(a) often fidgets with hands or feet or squirms in seat

(b) often leaves seat in classroom or in other situations in which remaining seated is expected

(c) often runs about or climbs excessively in situations in which it is inappropriate (in adolescents or adults, may be limited to subjective feelings of restlessness)

(d) often has difficulty playing or engaging in leisure activities quietly

(e) is often "on the go" or often acts as if "driven by a motor"

(f) often talks excessively

TABLE 3–1.	**DSM-IV-TR diagnostic criteria for attention-deficit/hyperactivity disorder** *(continued)*

Impulsivity

    (g) often blurts out answers before questions have been completed

    (h) often has difficulty awaiting turn

    (i) often interrupts or intrudes on others (e.g., butts into conversations or games)

B. Some hyperactive-impulsive or inattentive symptoms that caused impairment were present before age 7 years.

C. Some impairment from the symptoms is present in two or more settings (e.g., at school [or work] and at home).

D. There must be clear evidence of clinically significant impairment in social, academic, or occupational functioning.

E. The symptoms do not occur exclusively during the course of a pervasive developmental disorder, schizophrenia, or other psychotic disorder and are not better accounted for by another mental disorder (e.g., mood disorder, anxiety disorder, dissociative disorder, or a personality disorder).

Code based on type:

    314.01 Attention-deficit/hyperactivity disorder, combined type: if both criteria A1 and A2 are met for the past 6 months

    314.00 Attention-deficit/hyperactivity disorder, predominantly inattentive type: if criterion A1 is met but criterion A2 is not met for the past 6 months

    314.01 Attention-deficit/hyperactivity disorder, predominantly hyperactive-impulsive type: if criterion A2 is met but criterion A1 is not met for the past 6 months

Clinical skill, familiarity with normal development, and rigorous application of the diagnostic criteria are needed to diagnose ADHD, because inattention, impulsivity, and overactivity are common in children, especially boys. Children with ADHD may appear quite different to observers in different environments. Teachers expect more extended concentration and physical stillness than do parents. When the child is in a highly structured or novel setting, is engaged in a stimulating activity (e.g., a computer game), or is alone with an interested adult, symptoms may not be apparent at all, except in the most severe cases of ADHD. Symptoms typically worsen in situations that are unstructured, boring, and minimally supervised or that require sustained attention or mental effort. Problems, therefore, are often far more apparent to the teacher in a busy classroom than to the clinician in a quiet office. The clinical waiting area may provide a more realistic sample of behavior. Core deficits in ADHD include impairment relative to expected developmental level in learning and following rules (e.g., how to solve academic problems or how to behave in school and with friends) and difficulty in inhibiting impulsive responses to internal wishes or needs or to external attractions or provocations.

Many children with ADHD have high levels of motor activity in a variety of settings. When children are expected to be highly active (e.g., on the playground), children with and without ADHD have similar activity levels. In the classroom, however, restlessness, fidgeting, and walking or running around without permission cause problems. The child with ADHD often energetically explores new places and things. On entering a room, the child may immediately begin to touch and climb. He or she may inadvertently break things or hurt him- or herself or others.

Children with ADHD have great difficulty with motivation, sustained attention, organization, and completion when tasks are difficult, complex, long, or boring. These youngsters are unusually prone to seek immediate gratification. Resulting school problems include delayed learning, poor study skills, incomplete homework and tests with careless mistakes, and disruptive behavior. These problems may lead to erratic or failing grades, special class placement, suspension, expulsion, or dropping out.

Peers often perceive children with ADHD as immature and irritating and often avoid or neglect them because of their low frustration tolerance; difficulty following rules; and intrusive, bossy, and socially inappropriate behavior. Peers learn quickly that it is easy to tease children with ADHD or to set them up to get into trouble with adults.

Epidemiology

Prevalence estimates of ADHD vary, due to differences in diagnostic criteria, samples, and assessment methods. DSM-IV-TR cites a rate of 3%–7% in school-age children. Community surveys have found ADHD in as many as 17% of boys and 8% of girls of elementary school age and 11% of boys and 6% of girls in adolescence. A rigorous record-based birth cohort community study found a cumulative incidence by age 19 of 7.5% for definite ADHD (Barbaresi et al. 2002). ADHD is present in 30%–50% of child psychiatric outpatients and 40%–70% of child psychiatric inpatients, often in combination with other psychiatric disorders. In elementary school–age children, the boy-to-girl ratio is typically 9 to 1 in clinical settings but in community surveys is 2–3 to 1. Girls are more likely to have the predominantly inattentive type than the combined type, and, compared with boys, are less likely to have comorbid disruptive behavior disorders and more likely to have intellectual impairment and comorbid anxiety and depression. Although in most ways, boys and girls with ADHD are similar in symptoms, impairment, and response to treatment, girls with ADHD are less likely to be identified or receive treatment than are boys with the disorder.

ADHD has been found to exist in all countries where studies have been done. Greater reported prevalence in the United States appears to result from differing diagnostic practices and cultural expectations. Because all children in the United States are expected to attend school until age 18 years, academic and behavior problems are detected in youth who in other countries would no longer be in school.

Comorbidity

ADHD commonly occurs in association with other psychiatric disorders, particularly ODD and CD. As many as 50% of clinically referred children with ADHD also have CD, and many others have ODD; therefore, much of the ADHD literature is actually about the combination of ADHD plus ODD or CD. In clinical settings, approximately one-third of patients with ADHD also have a mood and/ or anxiety disorder. Although ADHD is very common in youth with

Tourette's disorder, relatively few children with ADHD also have Tourette's. The presence of ADHD not uncommonly complicates the clinical course of mental retardation and specific learning disorders. In adolescents, comorbid substance abuse is seen.

Etiology

ADHD is a heterogeneous syndrome, and various factors contribute to etiology. The common feature is relative dysfunction in the prefrontal cortex, which controls many "executive functions" such as planning, organization, and impulse control. One subgroup may have a predominantly genetic etiology, whereas in another, ADHD may be the result of biological environmental insults. Although school and home environment can influence the severity of ADHD symptoms, child-rearing practices do not cause ADHD.

A wide variety of biological findings reflect possible etiologies. Neurochemical studies of ADHD suggest that multiple neurotransmitter systems are involved, including norepinephrine and dopamine. Anatomic imaging studies have found that, as a group, children with ADHD show differences relative to control subjects in brain areas associated with executive functioning: smaller frontal lobe volume, delayed cortical development, different symmetry of basal ganglia regions, and smaller volume of the cerebellar vermis.

Imaging findings are not specific enough to be useful in the diagnosis of ADHD, only in ruling in or out a suspected neurological lesion. Functional magnetic resonance imaging (fMRI) offers promise in research on understanding the underlying brain mechanisms of attention and impulse control.

Genetics

The genetic contribution to the etiology of ADHD is substantial, with an average heritability of 75%–80%. In addition, children with ADHD without conduct problems are likely to have relatives with learning problems. Children with both ADHD and CD are more likely to have relatives with CD, adult antisocial behavior or personality, and substance abuse. Mood disorders are common in families with ADHD.

The hereditary component of ADHD is polygenic, rather than a single-gene defect. The specific mechanism of genetic transmission in ADHD has not been identified, although possibly contributing genes have been identified. In one prospective study, ADHD subjects with certain genes were more likely to develop aggression and other symptoms of CD (Caspi et al. 2008).

Medical Factors

Children with identifiable medical or neurological causes represent a small proportion of the ADHD population, and many children with medical risk factors do not have ADHD (Table 3–2).

Nonlocalizing neurological "soft signs" (e.g., clumsiness, left–right confusion, perceptual–motor dyscoordination, dysgraphia) are common in children with ADHD, but 15% of children without ADHD have as many as five soft signs, and children with anxiety disorders also have these signs. The presence or absence of soft signs, then, is not helpful in diagnosis but may identify target symptoms for treatment.

Course and Prognosis

Mothers of some youngsters with ADHD (especially those meeting hyperactive–impulsive criteria) recall excessive intrauterine kicking or report, "When he began to walk, he ran." Although ADHD can be diagnosed by age 3 years, considerable overlap with normal high activity level, impulsivity, limited frustration tolerance, and short attention span is found before age 5 years. Diagnosis is often delayed until elementary school, where expectations for physical stillness, prolonged attention, and conformity to social norms are greater and there is greater comparison to peers. Verbally skilled, nonoppositional children who do not have learning disabilities and who are not severely hyperactive may not be given a diagnosis until they experience the greater academic demands for organization and concentrated effort in middle school or high school, or even college or graduate school.

TABLE 3–2.	Medical contributions to attention-deficit/ hyperactivity disorder
Prenatal	Young mother Poor maternal health Maternal use of cigarettes or alcohol
Perinatal	Prematurity Postmaturity Intra-uterine growth retardation
Infancy	Malnutrition
Toxicity	Lead poisoning
Genetic disorders	Fragile X syndrome Glucose-6-phosphate dehydrogenase deficiency Generalized resistance to thyroid hormone Phenylketonuria
Brain injury	Trauma Infection

ADHD is not a benign or self-limited childhood disorder; it has a chronic or even lifelong course. As children mature, physical hyperactivity typically decreases. However, in adolescence, most continue to be symptomatic. As many as 30%–50% of clinically diagnosed hyperactive children continue to have the diagnosis of ADHD in adulthood, and other young adults have some symptoms of ADHD with impaired functioning. Secondary effects include low self-esteem and significantly compromised social skills. These individuals have more school failure, car accidents, changes in residence, court appearances, suicide attempts, early sexual activity, and problems with relationships than do young adults without ADHD. Children with ADHD are at increased risk for substance abuse or delinquency as adolescents only if they also had CD in childhood. "Pure" ADHD may increase the risk for substance abuse disorders in adulthood, however (Charach et al. 2011). ADHD also increases risk of cigarette smoking, including earlier onset and more difficulty quitting. Comorbid ADHD and CD in childhood also predict antisocial behavior and antisocial personality disorder in adolescence and adulthood. The absence of significant conduct problems or defiant, aggressive behavior toward adults in childhood predicts a better prognosis for ADHD. Childhood comorbid anxiety or mood disorders tend to persist (Biederman et al. 1996).

Parental responses to children with ADHD can aggravate or improve the course of the child's illness. Observation studies indicate that mothers tend to have more controlling, directive, structure-setting, and negative responses to their children with ADHD than control mothers have to their children (Tallmadge and Barkley 1983). Interestingly, when the ADHD child's behavior is improved by stimulant medication, the parents become more positive and less controlling (Tallmadge and Barkley 1983). Much of the parent–child conflict appears to be caused by comorbid ODD rather than by the ADHD per se. Children with ADHD are often more compliant with their fathers' requests than with their mothers'. Living with a child who has ADHD, especially one who also has CD or ODD, can push parents and siblings beyond the point at which they can cope adaptively with the stress. Given the strong genetic contribution to ADHD, it is not uncommon for one or both parents to be struggling to master their own inattention and impulsivity. ADHD provides an example of how an early-onset disorder, often with a genetic or neurological etiology, can be modified by life experiences and developmental processes, including educational programming; neighborhood supports; individual compensatory strengths such as easy temperament, engaging personality, athletic abilities, and intelligence; and family emotional, social, and financial resources.

Evaluation

Children and adolescents with ADHD commonly do not admit to symptoms of hyperactivity, inattention, and impulsivity. The patient interview is useful, nonetheless, for the clinician to observe the child's behavior and to identify any comorbid psychiatric disorders.

The parent interview is crucial for both ADHD diagnosis and more comprehensive assessment. Key parts of the history include obstetrical history (e.g., maternal substance use, prenatal or perinatal injury), medical history (e.g., seizures, thyroid disorder, head trauma, tics, medication use), screening questions for sleep disorders (e.g., loud snoring), traumatic events (including neglect or abuse), family residence (e.g., lead exposure from paint or exhaust fumes), family psychiatric history, family medical history (e.g., thyroid disorder), and any factors that may increase the risk of medication abuse by the child, siblings, or parents. Special emphasis is placed on school reports of grades, learning, and behavior (including behavior on the school bus and in the cafeteria). Normed parent and teacher rating scales are key—either general ones like the Child Behavior Checklist (CBCL) and the Teacher Report Form (TRF) (see Chapter 2) or DSM-IV-TR–based symptom ratings such as the Child Symptom Inventory or SNAP-IV (rating form and scoring instructions available at http://adhd.net).

The physical examination should include possible signs of physical anomalies, thyroid disorder, or chronic illness, as well as baseline findings relevant to subsequent medication treatment such as height and weight, tics, and cardiac status. Neurological examination or tests (e.g., electroencephalogram [EEG] or brain scan) are indicated only in the presence of focal neurological signs or clinical suggestions of a seizure disorder or a decline in neurological functioning. Acuity of vision and hearing should be tested. Laboratory measurement of thyroid function or blood lead level (and possibly free erythrocyte protoporphyrin) is indicated only if suggested by history or physical examination. A baseline electrocardiogram (ECG) is indicated prior to medication treatment only if patient history or examination or family history finds cardiac risk factors.

Psychological testing is useful to assess intellectual ability, academic achievement, and possible specific learning disorders. Although observations during testing may provide data on attention, distractibility, impulsivity, ability to stay seated, and frustration tolerance, a normal performance on individual testing does not preclude the diagnosis of ADHD. Neuropsychological evaluation may be requested to evaluate specific deficits suggested by history, physical examination, or basic psychological testing. Speech and language evaluation may be needed.

ADHD is a clinical diagnosis made on the basis of interviews and standardized parent and teacher behavior rating scales. EEG, brain imaging, laboratory tests, psychological tests, and computerized tests of vigilance are not diagnostic for ADHD.

Differential Diagnosis

Because the usual long-term course of ADHD is gradual improvement, sustained worsening behavior (apart from periods of environmental stress) suggests the emergence of a different psychiatric disorder. A positive treatment response to stimulant medication does not confirm a diagnosis of ADHD or eliminate another diagnosis. Clinical expertise is necessary to differentiate ADHD from *normal high activity level*. Problems of recent onset and brief duration may represent an *adjustment disorder*. For a diagnosis of ADHD, some symptoms causing impairment must have been present before age 7 years, and criteria must have been met for at least the past 6 months.

Various *physical problems* (medical disorders, sleep disorders, or lack of adequate sleep or nutrition) can interfere with attention. Hyper- or hypothyroidism, as well as the effects of prescribed medications or the abuse of drugs, can mimic ADHD. In addition, *situational anxiety, child abuse or neglect, posttraumatic stress disorder,* or *boredom in school* can present with inattention, hyperactivity, or impulsivity. *CD* and *ODD* are characterized by deliberate or provocative noncompliance, as distinguished from the impulsive or inattentive failure to comply seen in ADHD, although these disorders often occur with ADHD. *Depression* or *anxiety* may present with deficits in attention. Anxious children may appear fidgety and restless, but they can verbalize worries or fears. Symptoms of anxiety are most apparent in new situations, whereas ADHD typically worsens with increased familiarity. *Mania* or *bipolar mixed state* may take uncharacteristic forms in prepubertal children and should be considered, especially in patients with a family history of bipolar disorder. *Mood disorders* are generally more episodic than ADHD and have prominent symptoms of sadness or hypomania.

Accurate differential diagnosis is particularly crucial to rule out *psychosis,* because stimulant treatment can exacerbate psychotic symptoms and disorganization. Children with ADHD do not have hallucinations, delusions, or formal thought disorder. However, distractibility and excessive talking may resemble "loose" thought patterns, and impulsivity may lead to potentially dangerous behavior and a lack of awareness of the environment that may be confused with poor reality testing. Children with *pervasive developmental disorder* (PDD) often show hyperactivity, inattention, and impulsivity, but a diagnosis in the PDD category (including autistic disorder) preempts a diagnosis of ADHD. Children with undiagnosed *mental retardation* or *learning disorders* are often mistakenly referred for stimulant treatment because of inattention, distractibility, and inability to follow directions in school.

Monitoring Treatment

Treatment outcome is best evaluated by the reports of caregivers in various settings. Regular reports on behavior and academic progress from teachers and other observers are useful. Brief rating scales completed by teachers weekly during dose titration and at intervals thereafter are an efficient means of gathering school-related information. The items on the Child Attention Problems (CAP) Rating Scale (Barkley 1990) are similar to many of the DSM-IV-TR symptoms of ADHD (Table 3–3). Scoring of inattention and overactivity is based on a large normative sample (Table 3–4).

The IOWA Conners Teacher Rating Scale is a short report form for treatment monitoring that covers both ADHD symptoms and defiance or oppositional behavior (Loney and Milich 1982; Pelham et al. 1989). Some investigators and clinicians use computerized laboratory tests of attention, vigilance, and impulsivity, such as the Continuous Performance Test (CPT), to assess medication effect.

TABLE 3–3.   **Child Attention Problems (CAP) Rating Scale**

Child's name: _____   Child's age:_____

Today's date: _____   Child's sex: Male ❏

                                                  Female ❏

Filled out by: _____

Below is a list of items that describes pupils. For each item that describes
the pupil now or within the past week, check whether the item is Not true,
Somewhat or sometimes true, or Very or often true. Please check all items
as well as you can, even if some do not seem to apply to this pupil.

	Not true	Somewhat or sometimes true	Very or often true
1. Fails to finish things he/she starts	❏	❏	❏
2. Can't concentrate, can't pay attention for long	❏	❏	❏
3. Can't sit still, restless, or hyperactive	❏	❏	❏
4. Fidgets	❏	❏	❏
5. Daydreams or gets lost in his/her thoughts	❏	❏	❏
6. Impulsive or acts without thinking	❏	❏	❏
7. Difficulty following directions	❏	❏	❏
8. Talks out of turn	❏	❏	❏
9. Messy work	❏	❏	❏
10. Inattentive, easily distracted	❏	❏	❏
11. Talks too much	❏	❏	❏
12. Fails to carry out assigned tasks	❏	❏	❏

Please feel free to write any comments about the pupil's work or behavior
in the last week.

Source.   Reprinted with permission from Craig Edelbrock, Ph.D., 1967. (In the
public domain; may be reproduced but not changed or sold.) Available on the Internet at http://www.dbpeds.org/pdf/cap.pdf.

TABLE 3–4.   **Child Attention Problems (CAP) Rating Scale scoring**

Each of the 12 items is scored 0, 1, or 2.
Total score: Sum of the scores on all items
Subscores:
   Inattention: Sum of scores on items 1, 2, 5, 7, 9, 10, and 12
   Overactivity: Sum of scores on items 3, 4, 6, 8, and 11
Scores recommended as the upper limit of the normal range (93rd percentile):

	Boys		**Girls**	
Age (years)	6–11	12–16	6–11	12–16
Inattention	9	9	8	7
Overactivity	6	7	5	4
Total score	15	16	13	11

Source.   Personal communication, Craig Edelbrock, Ph.D., 1986. Scoring form available on the Internet at http://www.dbpeds.org/pdf/capscore.pdf.

Because these tests measure a limited domain of performance in an artificial environment, they should not be substituted for clinical judgment based on the reports of observers in different settings. Behavioral observations and measurement of productivity and accuracy on timed samples of reading or math problems are more ecologically valid.

Treatment

The cornerstones of treatment are education about the disorder, appropriate school and class placement and academic remediation (if necessary), and medication treatment. Mild cases of ADHD may respond to parent education, behavior modification, and school consultation alone, especially in young children. If medication and environmental modification do not lead to sufficiently improved behavior, academic performance, and social adjustment, or if co-morbid psychiatric conditions are present, then additional treatments should be considered, based on the specific problems of the child and family.

Parent Education

Education of parents regarding the nature of the disorder and its management is key to the treatment of ADHD. Efficient parent education methods include parent groups in the clinical setting, books (see Appendix), and referral to a support group such as CHADD (Children and Adults With Attention-Deficit/Hyperactivity Disorder) (see Appendix). Parents are taught to manage the child's environment by providing consistent routines and structure, reducing excessive stimulation, and averting predictable opportunity for misbehavior. At home, parents are advised to establish specific spaces for homework, remove easily damaged furnishings, closely monitor peer activities, and avoid taking the child to supermarkets and shopping malls. Parents can be coached on how best to work with the school to meet their child's needs.

School-Related Interventions

Special education is not always required but is useful for many patients with ADHD. The clinician may assess the need for special services after the child is receiving the maximum benefit from medication. The parent (and the clinician, with parental permission) should inform school officials about the child's vulnerabilities and strengths. Regular reports from the teacher on behavior and academic performance are essential for best outcome. An Individualized Education Program (IEP) or a 504 plan can be developed with the school to ensure that the child will receive needed services.

Useful and practical adaptations by teachers include consistent classroom structure and routines, seating the child near the teacher and away from disruptive peers or distractions, dividing assignments into small segments, reducing the quantity of repetitive classwork or homework, and communicating consistently with parents. A notebook for documenting assignment and completion of homework that is carried daily between teacher and parent can be effective. The Daily

Report Card (see Chapter 9) targets specific behaviors, and can be completed by the teacher with consequences provided by the parent. Closely supervised recess, physical education, bus, and cafeteria arrangements are sometimes needed. If these modifications are not sufficient, a small and perhaps self-contained classroom or resource room with a high teacher-to-student ratio, one-to-one tutoring, or remediation of specific learning disorders can be beneficial.

Academic transitions require careful planning. The move from elementary school, with smaller classes and fewer teachers, to middle school and then to high school is often very difficult for youngsters with ADHD. The decrease in structure and supervision along with the increased expectations for autonomous functioning and organization may result in dramatic exacerbation of academic and behavior problems.

Pharmacotherapy

Medication is the primary treatment for the core symptoms of ADHD. The vast majority of children with ADHD have a positive response to one or more drugs. Unfortunately, despite more than 50 years of research, specific predictors of response to one or all psychostimulants have not been demonstrated. Dosage titration requires individual tailoring to optimize behavior and learning in different settings throughout the day. Drug treatment may continue for years, with periodic dose adjustments needed. A few patients no longer need treatment by adolescence, but many individuals require medication through adolescence and into adulthood.

Prevalence of medication prescription for ADHD varies widely among communities. Medications appear to be underused in some areas, especially when schools and parents have difficulty accessing diagnostic and treatment resources. In some medical practices, however, medications may be prescribed too freely, with insufficient evaluation and follow-up. Specific medications and their use are covered in Chapter 8.

The psychostimulants methylphenidate and amphetamine (and related compounds; see Table 8–1) are the most established pharmacological agents in child psychiatry; their short-term clinical effectiveness and safety have been confirmed in more than 100 double-blind studies. A stimulant medication is the first-line drug for ADHD, with one class being tried if the other fails. The second-line choice is atomoxetine (Strattera), a norepinephrine reuptake inhibitor that has an FDA indication for ADHD. The α-adrenergic agonists guanfacine and clonidine have long been used "off-label" in the treatment of ADHD, as third-line single agents or supplements to stimulants, but recently, long-acting forms of guanfacine (Intuniv) and clonidine (Kapvay) have received FDA approval for indications in pediatric ADHD. At the end of the algorithm would be the antidepressant bupropion (which has supporting research in ADHD but does not have an FDA indication). Modafinil, a nonstimulant wake-promoting agent approved for treatment of narcolepsy, is used occasionally (especially by neurologists). When comorbid aggression is not manageable with optimal use of the above medications plus behavioral therapy, cautious adjunctive use of an atypical antipsychotic may be needed. If there is comorbid depression or anxiety, additional specific medications may be needed.

Psychotherapeutic Interventions

Behavior modification can improve academic achievement, reduce specifically targeted behavior problems, and decrease symptoms that are not helped by stimulants. Both punishment (time-out and response cost) and contingent rewards are required, and consistent, intensive, and prolonged (months to years) treatment may be needed. Response cost is the removal of points, rewards, or privileges following misbehavior as specified in a behavior modification plan. Parents and teachers must learn the specific techniques and be willing to invest the time and energy to implement them. Stimulants and behavior modification at home and at school may have separate and additive effects on motor behavior, attention and learning, and social functioning. Generalization and maintenance of improvement is unfortunately limited. Children may need to be taught social skills before behavior modification or medication can improve peer relationships. In a highly structured program (often not feasible to implement or maintain, however), the behavior of children with ADHD can be nearly normalized, but 30%–60% will improve further with the addition of a low dose of stimulant medication.

Cognitive-behavior therapy, in which children learn social and academic problem-solving strategies, monitor their own performance, remind themselves of rules, and praise themselves for accomplishments, generally is not effective in reducing ADHD symptoms, most likely because the child rarely uses the learned skills unless he or she is specifically cued by an adult. Individual psychotherapy may be useful to address comorbid disorders or sequelae of trauma, not core symptoms of ADHD. Family psychotherapy may reduce the conflict that results from raising a child with ADHD or may address primary marital dysfunction. Group therapy provides a setting where youth social skills deficits can be observed and remediated.

Unestablished Treatments

Dietary treatments remain popular with some families despite the minimal evidence of efficacy and the difficulty complying with special diets. Research on the Feingold diet (which omits natural and artificial salicylates and food dyes) is inconclusive, but elimination of food dyes might be helpful for a subgroup (5%) of children with ADHD, particularly those younger than 6 years. Double-blind studies do not confirm parents' reports of acute effects of food dyes. Even for those few children whose condition improves with a restricted diet, stimulants are a more potent treatment than diet. Despite anecdotal reports, there is no scientific evidence that sugar, food allergies, gluten, herbal remedies, yeast, trace minerals, or megavitamins influence the etiology or treatment of ADHD. Systemic reactions (irritability, fatigue) due to a variety of allergies or deficiencies or excesses in food intake may affect behavior and attention in some children. Some nonprofessionals have recommended caffeine as a more "natural" treatment of hyperactivity, but studies have found significant side effects and no evidence of efficacy.

Other unproven treatments that have enthusiastic advocates (often with financial interests) include anti–*Candida albicans* medication, neurotherapy (biofeedback training of brain waves), sensory integrative training, optometric vision training, chiropractic manipulation, metronome therapy, herbal regimens, homeopathy, massage, and acupuncture.

■ CONDUCT DISORDER

Clinical Description

Children and adolescents with CD repeatedly violate important societal rules or the personal rights of others (Table 3–5). The division of youths with CD into subgroups has been controversial. Those who behave aggressively may be differentiated from those who engage primarily in covert, nonconfrontational problem behaviors (e.g., stealing and truancy). In addition, whether aggressive behavior is "predatory" (goal oriented, planned) or "affective" (impulsive, reactive) may have implications for etiology and treatment.

DSM-IV-TR specifies two types of CD: childhood onset, in which at least one criterion is met before age 10 years, and adolescent onset. Longitudinal studies (Langbehn et al. 1998) have found that childhood onset is associated with male predominance, more physical aggression, impaired peer relationships, and comorbid ADHD. A typical course for this subtype is ODD in early childhood, which develops into full-blown CD by puberty, followed by risk of persistent CD and development of adult antisocial personality disorder. Those with adolescent onset have few symptoms before puberty and are less likely to be aggressive and more likely to be female than those in the early-onset group. Most of those with adolescent onset have friends but often in the context of a gang or other delinquent peer group. The prognosis for cessation of conduct problems is better if onset is in adolescence; however, course and outcome may be influenced by the nature of the delinquent group and the availability of alternative social supports.

Consequences of truancy and suspensions for violating school rules, as well as coexisting attention problems and specific learning disorders, include loss of interest in school, school failure and drop-

TABLE 3–5. **DSM-IV-TR diagnostic criteria for conduct disorder**

A. A repetitive and persistent pattern of behavior in which the basic rights of others or major age-appropriate societal norms or rules are violated, as manifested by the presence of three (or more) of the following criteria in the past 12 months, with at least one criterion present in the past 6 months:

Aggression to people and animals
(1) often bullies, threatens, or intimidates others
(2) often initiates physical fights
(3) has used a weapon that can cause serious physical harm to others (e.g., a bat, brick, broken bottle, knife, gun)
(4) has been physically cruel to people
(5) has been physically cruel to animals
(6) has stolen while confronting a victim (e.g., mugging, purse snatching, extortion, armed robbery)
(7) has forced someone into sexual activity

Destruction of property
(8) has deliberately engaged in fire setting with the intention of causing serious damage
(9) has deliberately destroyed others' property (other than by fire setting)

Deceitfulness or theft
(10) has broken into someone else's house, building, or car
(11) often lies to obtain goods or favors or to avoid obligations (i.e., "cons" others)
(12) has stolen items of nontrivial value without confronting a victim (e.g., shoplifting, but without breaking and entering; forgery)

Serious violations of rules
(13) often stays out at night despite parental prohibitions, beginning before age 13 years
(14) has run away from home overnight at least twice while living in parental or parental surrogate home (or once without returning for a lengthy period)
(15) is often truant from school, beginning before age 13 years

B. The disturbance in behavior causes clinically significant impairment in social, academic, or occupational functioning.

TABLE 3–5.	**DSM-IV-TR diagnostic criteria for conduct disorder** *(continued)*

C. If the individual is age 18 years or older, criteria are not met for antisocial personality disorder.

> *Code* based on age at onset:
>
>> **312.81   Conduct disorder, childhood-onset type:**   onset of at least one criterion characteristic of conduct disorder prior to age 10 years
>>
>> **312.82   Conduct disorder, adolescent-onset type:**   absence of any criteria characteristic of conduct disorder prior to age 10 years
>>
>> **312.89   Conduct disorder, unspecified onset:**   age at onset is not known

out, and eventual unemployment. Youths with CD are at increased medical risk for early pregnancy; sexually transmitted diseases; physical injury from fighting, accidents, rape, or even murder; and the sequelae of smoking, drinking, and drug abuse. Rates of suicidal ideation and behavior are increased, especially when substance use is present.

Despite heterogeneity among youth with CD, certain psychological characteristics are common (Table 3–6).

Epidemiology

DSM-IV-TR cites prevalence estimates of CD among children and adolescents in the United States ranging from less than 1% to more than 10%. Although the prevalence of CD in girls has increased, boys still outnumber girls by 3–4:1. Less is known about CD in girls than in boys. Boys commit far more violent crimes than girls do (8:1). When self-report data are used, the overall prevalence of misconduct and delinquent behaviors increases, and the male predominance for crime declines to about 2:1. Cultural attitudes toward gender, race, and class may affect the relative likelihood of a youth's being identified as having a CD. CD is frequent among youths referred to outpatient psychiatric services.

TABLE 3–6. **Common psychological characteristics of children and adolescents with conduct disorder**

Attention deficits, low frustration tolerance

Impulsivity, recklessness

Learning disorders, especially in reading

Negative mood
Sullenness
Irritability
Volatile anger

Low self-esteem

Impaired cognitions
Distortions of size and time awareness
Lack of or distorted connection between prior events and consequences
Limited ability to generate, evaluate, and implement alternative problem-solving strategies

Emotional deficits
Minimization of fear and sadness, exaggeration of anger
Lack of empathy
Lack of guilt

Impaired interpersonal relations
Suspiciousness, with cognitive distortions
Attributional bias: misperception of others' actions as hostile
Preference for nonverbal, action-oriented, aggressive solutions to problems
Callousness

Comorbidity

Comorbid psychiatric or neurological disorders are common in association with CD and contribute to its severity and chronicity. ADHD occurs in as many as half of children with CD in community surveys. In psychiatric clinical programs, CD without ADHD is rare. Posttraumatic stress disorder (PTSD) and dissociative disorders are often reported, especially by incarcerated delinquent youth. Hypervigilance, irritability, and flashbacks may contribute to aggression when youths feel threatened. Learning disorders (especially reading disorder and expressive language disorder) are common. Depression or bipolar disorder may be seen. Although it seems contradictory, anxiety and mood disorders are found in many youth with CD, especially girls, at increased rates after puberty. Substance use is often present and may not be recognized. Drug or alcohol use can aggravate impulsivity, risk taking, aggression, suicidality, and school failure.

Etiology

Many etiological factors have been implicated in the development of CD, which is a heterogeneous disorder (Table 3–7). Understanding the contributing factors for the individual patient is important in planning treatment. Current views emphasize an interaction among socioeconomic, cultural, family dynamic, temperamental, genetic, neurobiological, and psychiatric factors to explain the development and persistence of CD and its pattern of transmission from one generation to the next.

Data from a study of male twins suggest that, compared with adult antisocial behavior, juvenile conduct problems are more strongly related to environmental factors and less strongly related to genetic factors (Lyons et al. 1995). The interaction of inadequate and often abusive parenting with characteristics intrinsic to the child results in noncompliant and aggressive behaviors and deficient academic and social skills. Temperamental characteristics such as negative emotions, intense reactions, and inflexibility are associated with higher risk of CD. Multiple studies have found that birth complications combined with early maternal rejection (unwanted pregnancy, attempt to abort fetus, and placement outside the home before age 1 year), poor parenting, and parental mental illness increase the likelihood of violent criminal behavior (Raine 2002). Patterson and colleagues (1989) emphasized the importance of a parent–child negative spiral of ever-increasing aversive and coercive behaviors. In effect, these children train their parents to use harsh but inconsistent discipline, and the parents train the children in noncompliant, defiant, and antisocial behaviors. Although less is known about girls with CD, some data suggest that their families are even more dysfunctional than those of boys

TABLE 3–7.   **Factors implicated in the etiology of conduct disorders**

Genetic transmission of predisposing psychiatric disorder
   Antisocial personality disorder
   Oppositional defiant disorder
   Attention-deficit/hyperactivity disorder
   Substance abuse
   Mood disorders
   Learning disorders

Neurobiological
   Low autonomic activity/arousal (as shown by low resting heart rate)
   Intrauterine exposure to alcohol
   Maternal smoking (may be correlate or cause)
   Birth complications, low birth weight
   Head injuries from accidents or abuse

Temperament
   Difficult
      Resistant to parental discipline
      Poor adaptability to change
      Intense activity
   High level of novelty-seeking (may relate to dopamine D_4 receptor gene)

Other psychiatric disorders
   Posttraumatic stress disorder
   Communication disorders
   Psychosis, paranoia

Parenting characteristics
   Large family
   Young mother
   Absent or alcoholic father
   Conflict between parents
   Depressed, irritable, substance-using, or psychotic parent
   Lack of parental monitoring; inadequate supervision and limit setting
   Harsh and inconsistent, unpredictable discipline
   Rejection, abandonment, or neglect by parents
   Physical or sexual abuse
   Modeling of impulsivity, aggression, or antisocial behavior

TABLE 3–7.	**Factors implicated in the etiology of conduct disorders** *(continued)*

Parenting characteristics *(continued)*
  Lack of enculturation to use of language for problem-solving or to values of larger society
  Placement outside of the home as an infant or toddler
Social problems
  Poverty and cultural disadvantage
  Cultural behavior norms: gang- and drug-infested neighborhoods
  Rejection by prosocial peers
  Association with antisocial peers
  Early puberty (for girls only)

with CD. Rejection by peers and school failure encourage affiliation with similarly troubled peers. One study found that approximately one-third of prepubertal children with depressive mood disorders developed a DSM-III diagnosis of CD by age 19 years (Kovacs et al. 1988).

The multiple risk factors appear to have a cumulative effect. Most children with risk factors do not, however, develop CD. Divorce does not appear to be a major risk factor; family discord rather than separation appears to mediate the risk for CD. Protective factors are not well understood, but an easy or behaviorally inhibited temperament, areas of competence, adequate supervision at home, or a good relationship with one parent or another adult can reduce an at-risk child's chance of developing CD. Associating with nondelinquent peers and attending a school with a positive environment also offer some protection.

Course and Prognosis

The first signs of behavior problems—aggression, impulsivity, and noncompliance—may be seen as early as age 4 years. Several studies have found that the combination of aggression and shyness in first grade predicts adolescent delinquency and substance abuse. Symptoms tend to emerge in a predictable developmental sequence, with milder behaviors followed by more severe ones. Progression may stop at any stage. Early onset; greater frequency, number, and variety of conduct symptoms; and comorbid ADHD are associated with more severe and prolonged CD.

CD remits in many youths, but some lead lives of delinquency or develop antisocial personality disorder. Low IQ score and parental antisocial personality disorder predict persistence of CD (Loeber et al. 1995). A relatively small number of chronic offenders account for most juvenile crime. Recidivists are more likely to have early onset, poor school grades, and low socioeconomic status. In a 7-year follow-up of clinic-referred boys ages 7–12 years with CD, the majority showed fluctuating or increasing CD behaviors. At baseline, the minority with a more positive outcome were more likely to have lower severity of CD, fewer symptoms of ADHD, higher verbal IQ, greater family socioeconomic advantage, and biological parents who were not antisocial. Treatment or incarceration did not account for improvement (Lahey et al. 2002).

Despite the high risk for major psychiatric symptoms, substance abuse, functional impairment, and incarceration, many children with CD achieve a favorable adult adjustment. More adaptive social skills, more positive peer experiences, and adolescent onset predict a better long-term outcome. Innovative early childhood programs have been able to reduce delinquent outcomes and improve academic achievement in children at risk for CD, but successful model programs are rarely replicated or disseminated.

Evaluation

Youths with more severe and complex forms of CD require a comprehensive biopsychosocial evaluation by a multidisciplinary team that might include a child and adolescent psychiatrist, a clinical psychologist, a social worker, a pediatrician or specialist in adolescent medicine, a neurologist, an educational diagnostician and school consultant, a speech and language pathologist, occupational and recreational therapists, a legal advisor, and a case manager or probation officer.

Conventional diagnostic interviews may be difficult, because many youths with CD are uncomfortable or hostile when talking with adults in roles of authority and have a limited ability to express themselves verbally and to think abstractly. Efforts to establish rapport and careful questioning are essential to identify comorbid psychiatric disorders or neurological impairment. Patients often underreport deviant behaviors as a result of either unconscious denial or lying to avoid punishment. Sources of information in addition to the patient are essential. Youths generally report more of their covert behaviors, such as lying, stealing, vandalism, and fire setting, whereas parents are more likely to report their child's overt behaviors, such as aggression. However, parents who are trying to shield their child from legal consequences may not disclose behaviors.

Medical evaluation (especially in adolescents) should consider pregnancy, sexually transmitted diseases, and hepatitis, as well as any untreated medical disorder and a urine screen for abused drugs. Evaluation of neurological history is needed because of the frequency of head trauma (both contributing to and resulting from the CD) and seizures. Cognitive and educational assessment are indicated because of the high association with specific learning disorders and borderline intellectual functioning or mental retardation. In addition, truancy, comorbid ADHD, and lack of socialization to the value and culture of school may contribute to educational deficits.

Differential Diagnosis

CD is a heterogeneous descriptive diagnosis that is made if the symptoms meet the behavioral criteria. Because virtually any psychiatric disorder can present with disturbance of conduct, the clinician must evaluate the full range of Axis I psychiatric diagnoses, intelligence, neuropsychological performance, language and speech abilities, social competence, and family functioning. During an episode of depression or mania in *bipolar disorder,* irritability and impaired judgment can lead to behavior problems that can be distinguished from primary CD by their time course and associated mood symptoms. *Psychosis* in children and adolescents may result in behaviors consistent with CD. Differential diagnosis also includes *intermittent explosive disorder* and a spectrum of less severe disorders: *ODD, adjustment disorder with disturbance of conduct,* and child or adolescent *antisocial behavior* (a DSM-IV-TR V code), as well as typical mischief. Although many cases of CD (especially childhood onset) also meet criteria for ODD, DSM-IV-TR specifies that a diagnosis of ODD is preempted if criteria for CD are met.

Treatment

Despite the cost of CD to individuals, families, and society, few treatments with proven efficacy are available. The patient is rarely motivated to change, and the family and social environments may lack the necessary resources. Early-onset CD becomes increasingly resistant to treatment as the child enters adolescence; therefore, early intervention with young children is crucial. Treatment may take a variety of forms: family interventions, social support, behavior modification, psychopharmacology, or legal sanctions. The treatment setting may be the home; a school, clinic, hospital, or residential treatment program; or a specialized delinquency program. Complex cases of CD often require lengthy multimodal therapeutic interventions. The environment in which the patient is living or to which he or she will return must be considered. Comorbid conditions also require attention.

A containment structure and effective limit setting must be established quickly to provide a safe and stable environment for treatment. Limit setting at home may be compromised by parental conflict, parental absence, inconsistent discipline, vague or low expectations for appropriate behavior, or parental depression or other psychiatric illness. Creating or reinforcing limits for the child with CD may require counseling of parents, treatment of parents' psychiatric problems, increased supervision at home, surveillance at school, or use of legal mechanisms. Guardianship, hearings before judges, supervision by parole officers, or brief incarceration may be required for effective limit setting and communicating the significance of behavioral violations. Families may need concrete assistance with income, housing, legal matters, or medical care. If there are comorbid psychiatric disorders, hospitalizing the youth briefly may be useful for containment and intensive evaluation, perhaps including a trial of medication. More stringent criteria for "medical necessity" have decreased the frequency of hospitalization for pure form CD, in part because hospitalization is not effective as definitive treatment.

Psychotherapeutic Interventions

Several treatments based on behavioral and family systems principles have shown efficacy, when youth and families can be motivated to participate in and complete treatment programs. Even with treatment, many remain outside the normal range of problem behavior, however.

Parent management training (PMT) and functional family therapy (FFT) can be helpful for relatively motivated and intact families. Principles of behavior modification and family systems theory are used to improve communication and negotiation skills, encourage positive reinforcement, correct dysfunctional parent–child interaction patterns, and promote more effective and less damaging methods of discipline. Long-term positive effects have not been shown, however. Younger children are more likely than adolescents to benefit from parent training interventions. Multisystemic therapy (MST) (see Henggeler et al. 2009 in "Additional Reading"), a comprehensive treatment combining home-based systemic family therapy with behavior modification and direct intervention into the youth's social system, has been shown to be an effective treatment of delinquency in youths, even those from chaotic, multiproblem families; it improves adjustment of patients and family members and reduces future criminal behavior. The therapist empowers parents; enlists social service agencies; and actively reaches out into the home, school, and neighborhood. Individual supportive therapy or pharmacotherapy for the identified patient or a family member is added when necessary.

Group therapy, particularly in residential treatment or group-oriented facilities, uses peer pressure to promote positive change and to improve socialization skills. Caution is needed, because treating antisocial youth together in groups can lead to contagion and worsening of problem behaviors. Insight-oriented individual psychotherapy is not useful.

Pharmacotherapy

There is no medication treatment of CD, but treatment of comorbid disorder(s) can be useful (see Chapter 8). In patients with coexisting ADHD, stimulants can decrease impulsive conduct symptoms, verbal and physical aggression, overactivity, and inattention. Bupropion or guanfacine also may be effective.

CD that is secondary to a major depression may remit when the depression is successfully treated. Lithium may be considered in the treatment of severe impulsive aggression, especially when it is accompanied by explosive, irritable, labile affect. In a well-designed controlled study, lithium was shown to be equal or superior to haloperidol in reducing aggression, hostility, and tantrums and to have fewer side effects (Campbell et al. 1995). Lithium may be the first pharmacological choice if the patient with CD has a family history of bipolar disorder.

Patients who have severe impulsive aggression with emotional lability and irritability, an abnormal electroencephalogram, a strong clinical suggestion of epileptic phenomena, or nonresponse to lithium may benefit from a trial of carbamazepine or valproate. Antipsychotic medications may decrease aggressive symptoms that result from psychosis. Even in nonpsychotic, severely aggressive children, atypical antipsychotics such as risperidone may reduce aggression, hostility, negativism, and explosiveness, although the side-effect profile (cognitive dulling, weight gain and metabolic syndrome, and risk of tardive dyskinesia) may be problematic. Propranolol, a β-adrenergic blocker, may be useful in patients with otherwise uncontrollable rage reactions and impulsive aggression, especially those with evidence of organicity.

School and Juvenile Justice Interventions

School interventions include special attention to behavior control; individualized educational programming; vocational training; and remediation of language, speech, and other specific learning disorders. Despite their political popularity, "boot camps" are not effective in reducing future crimes committed by juvenile delinquents (Henggeler and Schoenwald 1994).

■ OPPOSITIONAL DEFIANT DISORDER

Clinical Description

ODD is considered to be the developmentally earlier, less severe form of disruptive behavior disorder. Children with ODD show argumentative, disobedient, and defiant behavior, without serious violation of the rights of other people. These children are stubborn, negativistic, and provocative. Anger-related symptoms are typically directed at parents and teachers. A lesser degree of anger dyscontrol may be seen in peer relationships.

DSM-IV-TR defines ODD as a pattern of negativistic, hostile, disobedient, and defiant behavior lasting at least 6 months, during which at least four of the behavioral criteria are present at a frequency greater than that typical for the child's age and developmental level. Data from a community survey provide guidance in determining when a behavior occurs more frequently than expected for age (Angold and Costello 1996). DSM-IV-TR symptom criteria and suggested cutoff frequencies are listed in Table 3–8. To diagnose ODD, the symptoms must not occur exclusively during the course of a psychotic or mood disorder.

A crucial feature of ODD is the self-defeating stand that these children take in arguments. They may be willing to lose something they want (a privilege or toy) rather than lose a battle or lose face. The oppositional struggle takes on a life of its own in the child's mind and becomes more important than the reality of the situation. The child may experience "rational" interventions as continuing arguments.

TABLE 3–8.	DSM-IV-TR criteria and suggested cutoff frequencies for oppositional defiant disorder

DSM-IV-TR symptom criteria	Suggested cutoff frequency
1. Often loses temper	Twice a week
2. Often argues with adults	Twice a week
3. Often actively defies or refuses to comply with adults' requests or rules	Twice a week
4. Often deliberately annoys people	Four times a week
5. Often blames others for his or her mistakes or misbehavior	Once in 3 months
6. Is often touchy or easily annoyed by others	Twice a week
7. Is often angry and resentful	Four times a week
8. Is often spiteful or vindictive	Once in 3 months

Source. American Psychiatric Association 2000; Angold and Costello 1996.

Disobedience can take the form of overt defiance and provocation or dawdling and procrastination, as well as "sneaky" behavior. Parents, and sometimes teachers, become exhausted, frustrated, and angry. As a result, discipline veers between overly punitive and hopelessly lax. By the time of clinical referral, the findings are the result of an interactive, negative spiral between parents and child.

Epidemiology

The changing criteria for ODD have prevented stable prevalence estimates. Perhaps 3%–15% of children have ODD, with equal or slightly higher rates in boys than girls. ODD is common in psychiatric clinics and in classes for children with emotional disturbances and learning disabilities. It often occurs concurrently with ADHD.

Etiology

Several psychosocial mechanisms have been hypothesized to contribute to ODD:

- Parents use inconsistent methods of disciplining, structuring, and limit setting.
- Children identify with a stubborn and impulsive parent who acts as a role model for oppositional and defiant interactions with other people.
- Parents have insufficient time and emotional energy for the child.

Marital problems are common in the parents of children with ODD, but it is difficult to distinguish the cause from the effect of raising such a child. Genetic, neurobiological, and temperamental factors may also contribute. The features of ODD and difficult temperament overlap significantly. One study of adopted high-risk youth suggests that symptoms of ODD in adolescent males may be linked to genetic traits leading to adult antisocial personality (Langbehn et al. 1998).

Course and Prognosis

Some children with ODD develop CD, but many do not. In one sample of 7- to 12-year-old clinic-referred boys with ODD, 44% developed CD over a 3-year period (Loeber et al. 1995). Risk factors for progression of ODD to CD include poverty and parental characteristics such as a mother who is young when her first child is born and parents who abuse substances, discipline children inconsistently, and supervise children inadequately. Risk factors in the child are low IQ, physical fighting, and resistance to parental discipline.

Evaluation and Differential Diagnosis

Psychiatric evaluation of the child and family is needed to rule out alternative or comorbid disorders and to seek family and psychosocial contributing factors. The ODD symptoms are generally reported by parents and caregivers. The children may not view themselves as defiant or argumentative and often blame parents, authority figures, and peers. Symptoms are more prominent when the child is with familiar people.

Although these behaviors can be normal for children in phases during toddlerhood and adolescence, the 6-month duration criterion for ODD ordinarily excludes these developmental phenomena. Some children are simply temperamentally stubborn but lack the pattern of more severe disturbance characteristic of ODD. Children with ODD are often annoying or spiteful but stop short of the pattern of serious behavior problems seen in CD. A diagnosis of CD precludes a diagnosis of ODD.

Severe *separation anxiety disorder, panic disorder,* or *obsessive-compulsive disorder* may lead to temper tantrums and dramatic resistance, but in these disorders the problem behavior is restricted to the feared situations, and in most cases these children can verbalize specific triggers of anxiety.

A key to the diagnosis of ODD is its lifelong pattern. Discrete periods of irritability and resistance to adult direction may be secondary to *major affective episodes* (depression or hypomania), *psychosis,* or an *adjustment disorder.* The intentional and provocative noncompliance characteristic of ODD should be differentiated from the noncompliance resulting from impulsivity and inattention in *ADHD,* although both disorders are often present. If criteria for both ODD and ADHD are met, both are diagnosed.

Oppositional behavior that is restricted to the school context may be a result of *mental retardation, borderline intelligence,* or a specific *developmental disorder* or lack of training in cultural norms and expectations.

Treatment

Multimodal programs such as Fast Track can reduce progression to CD in young children identified as at-risk (Conduct Problems Prevention Research Group 2002). PMT in behavior modification techniques such as positive reinforcement, giving more effective commands, "time-out," and token economies can reduce power struggles and modify oppositionality. Maximal improvement may result from combining the use of a social skills, problem-solving, and conflict management training group for the child with a behavior modification training group for parents (Webster-Stratton and Hammond 1997). Traditional individual or family systems psychotherapy is not helpful for the primary symptoms of ODD.

In children with coexisting ADHD, anxiety, or mood disorder, medication may reduce oppositional behavior and improve compliance.

■ REFERENCES

American Psychiatric Association: Diagnostic and Statistical Manual of Mental Disorders, 3rd Edition. Washington, DC, American Psychiatric Association, 1980

American Psychiatric Association: Diagnostic and Statistical Manual of Mental Disorders, 4th Edition, Text Revision. Washington, DC, American Psychiatric Association, 2000

Angold A, Costello EJ: Toward establishing an empirical basis for the diagnosis of oppositional defiant disorder. J Am Acad Child Adolesc Psychiatry 35:1205–1212, 1996

Barbaresi WJ, Katusic SK, Colligan RC, et al: How common is attention-deficit/hyperactivity disorder? Arch Pediatr Adolesc Med 156:217–224, 2002

Barkley RA: Attention Deficit Hyperactivity Disorder: A Handbook for Diagnosis and Treatment. New York, Guilford, 1990

Biederman J, Faraone S, Milberger S, et al: A prospective 4-year follow-up study of attention-deficit hyperactivity and related disorders. Arch Gen Psychiatry 53:437–446, 1996

Campbell M, Adams PB, Small AM, et al: Lithium in hospitalized aggressive children with conduct disorder: a double-blind and placebo-controlled study. J Am Acad Child Adolesc Psychiatry 34:445–453, 1995

Caspi A, Langley K, Milne B, et al: A replicated molecular genetic basis for subtyping antisocial behavior in children with ADHD. Arch Gen Psychiatry 65:203–210, 2008

Charach A, Yeung E, Climans T, et al: Childhood attention-deficit hyperactivity disorder and future substance use disorders: comparative meta-analyses. J Am Acad Child Adolesc Psychiatry 50:9–21, 2011

Conduct Problems Prevention Research Group: Evaluation of the first 3 years of the Fast Track prevention trial with children at high risk for adolescent conduct problems. J Abnorm Child Psychol 30:19–35, 2002

Henggeler SW, Schoenwald SK: Boot camps for juvenile offenders: just say no. Journal of Child and Family Studies 3:243–248, 1994

Kovacs M, Paulauskas S, Gatsonis C, et al: Depressive disorders in childhood, III: a longitudinal study of comorbidity with and risk for conduct disorders. J Affect Disord 15:205–217, 1988

Lahey BB, Loeber R, Burke J, et al: Adolescent outcomes of childhood conduct disorder among clinic-referred boys: predictors of improvement. J Abnorm Child Psychol 30:333–348, 2002

Langbehn DR, Cadoret RJ, Yates WR, et al: Distinct contributions of conduct and oppositional defiant symptoms to adult antisocial behavior: evidence from an adoption study. Arch Gen Psychiatry 55:821–829, 1998

Loeber R, Green SM, Keenan K, et al: Which boys will fare worse? Early predictors of the onset of conduct disorder in a six-year longitudinal study. J Am Acad Child Adolesc Psychiatry 34:499–509, 1995

Loney J, Milich R: Hyperactivity, inattention, and aggression in clinical practice. Advances in Developmental and Behavioral Pediatrics 3:113–147, 1982

Lyons MJ, True WR, Eisen SA, et al: Differential heritability of adult and juvenile antisocial traits. Arch Gen Psychiatry 52:906–915, 1995

Patterson GR, DeBaryshe BD, Ramsey E: A developmental perspective on antisocial behavior. Am Psychol 44:329–335, 1989

Pelham WE, Milich R, Murphy DA, et al: Normative data on the IOWA Conners Teacher Rating Scale. Journal of Clinical Child Psychology 18:259–262, 1989

Raine A: Biosocial studies of antisocial and violent behavior in children and adults: a review. J Abnorm Child Psychol 30:311–326, 2002

Tallmadge J, Barkley RA: The interactions of hyperactive and normal boys with their fathers and mothers. J Abnorm Child Psychol 11:565–579, 1983

Webster-Stratton C, Hammond M: Treating children with early-onset conduct problems: a comparison of child and parent training interventions. J Consult Clin Psychol 65:93–109, 1997

■ ADDITIONAL READING

American Academy of Child and Adolescent Psychiatry: Practice parameter for the assessment and treatment of children and adolescents with attention-deficit/hyperactivity disorder. J Am Acad Child Adolesc Psychiatry 46:894–921, 2007

American Academy of Child and Adolescent Psychiatry: Practice parameter for the assessment and treatment of children and adolescents with oppositional defiant disorder. J Am Acad Child Adolesc Psychiatry 46:126–141, 2007

Barkley RA: Attention-Deficit Hyperactivity Disorder: A Handbook for Diagnosis and Treatment, 3rd Edition. New York, Guilford, 2005

Henggeler SW, Schoenwald SK, Borduin CM, et al: Multisystemic Therapy for Antisocial Behavior in Children and Adolescents, 2nd Edition. New York, Guilford, 2009

Pliszka SR: Attention-deficit/hyperactivity disorder, in Dulcan's Textbook of Child and Adolescent Psychiatry. Edited by Dulcan MK. Washington, DC, American Psychiatric Publishing, 2010, pp 205–222

Thomas CR: Oppositional defiant disorder and conduct disorder, in Dulcan's Textbook of Child and Adolescent Psychiatry. Edited by Dulcan MK. Washington, DC, American Psychiatric Publishing, 2010, pp 223–240

4

OTHER AXIS I DISORDERS USUALLY FIRST DIAGNOSED IN INFANCY, CHILDHOOD, OR ADOLESCENCE

This chapter covers several disorders from the childhood-onset section of DSM-IV-TR (American Psychiatric Association 2000). These disorders always begin prior to adulthood, although they may not be diagnosed until later. Separation anxiety disorder, pica, rumination, encopresis, enuresis, and selective mutism nearly all remit by adulthood. Tourette's and other tic disorders typically become less severe by adulthood but may persist. Some children with reactive attachment disorder remain impaired in adulthood, but longitudinal studies have not been done.

■ SEPARATION ANXIETY DISORDER

Clinical Description

In separation anxiety disorder (SAD), cognitive, affective, somatic, and behavioral symptoms appear in response to genuine or fantasized separation from the individual(s) to whom the child is most attached. The key feature of SAD is excessive and age-inappropriate anxiety, fear, or worry concerning separation from home or primary attachment figures (Table 4–1). The anxiety can be experienced and expressed as an unrealistic fear of or worry about the child or parent being permanently separated from the other due to injury, kidnap-

---

TABLE 4–1.   **DSM-IV-TR diagnostic criteria for separation anxiety disorder**

A. Developmentally inappropriate and excessive anxiety concerning separation from home or from those to whom the individual is attached, as evidenced by three (or more) of the following:

  (1) recurrent excessive distress when separation from home or major attachment figures occurs or is anticipated
  (2) persistent and excessive worry about losing, or about possible harm befalling, major attachment figures
  (3) persistent and excessive worry that an untoward event will lead to separation from a major attachment figure (e.g., getting lost or being kidnapped)
  (4) persistent reluctance or refusal to go to school or elsewhere because of fear of separation
  (5) persistently and excessively fearful or reluctant to be alone or without major attachment figures at home or without significant adults in other settings
  (6) persistent reluctance or refusal to go to sleep without being near a major attachment figure or to sleep away from home
  (7) repeated nightmares involving the theme of separation
  (8) repeated complaints of physical symptoms (such as headaches, stomachaches, nausea, or vomiting) when separation from major attachment figures occurs or is anticipated

B. The duration of the disturbance is at least 4 weeks.
C. The onset is before age 18 years.
D. The disturbance causes clinically significant distress or impairment in social, academic (occupational), or other important areas of functioning.
E. The disturbance does not occur exclusively during the course of a pervasive developmental disorder, schizophrenia, or other psychotic disorder and, in adolescents and adults, is not better accounted for by panic disorder with agoraphobia.

---

ping, harm, or death. Symptoms can include nightmares with separation themes and inability to sleep alone, attend school, visit friends, go on errands, or stay at camp. In order to avoid leaving home, children with SAD will often complain of somatic symptoms such as stomachaches or headaches (which they may actually be experiencing) or report distressing events such as peers or teachers picking on them.

Not all children with school absenteeism have SAD, and not all children with SAD miss excessive amounts of school. However, school refusal often occurs within the context of psychiatric disorders, psychosocial vulnerabilities, impaired family functioning, parental psychopathology, and/or stressful life events. Approximately three-quarters of children with SAD exhibit school avoidance (Last et al. 1987). The historical term for school avoidance or school refusal secondary to SAD is *school phobia,* although this is not a DSM diagnosis. School absenteeism has various etiologies (Table 4–2). In a large clinical sample of children and adolescents with school refusal, 25% had both an anxiety and a depressive diagnosis, and half of the total group had either an anxiety or a depressive disorder (Bernstein et al. 1996).

TABLE 4–2.   **Causes of school absenteeism**

Separation anxiety disorder
Other psychiatric disorders
   Mood disorder
   Anxiety disorder
      Generalized anxiety disorder
      Phobic disorder (such as social phobia)
      Panic disorder
      Obsessive-compulsive disorder
   Psychotic disorder
Truancy (often associated with conduct disorder)
Substance abuse
Sociocultural conformity
   Permission granted by family (overt or covert)
   Normative peer behavior
Realistic fear
   Excessive teasing/humiliation or verbal harassment/bullying
   Physical bullying–intimidation or bodily harm
   Academic struggles or avoidance

Epidemiology

SAD has a reported prevalence of 3%–5% in youth (Black 1995; Shear et al. 2006), with higher prevalence in childhood compared with adolescence (Breton et al. 1999) and much higher rates of symptoms that do not meet full diagnostic criteria (Kashani and Orvaschel 1990). More recent research has shown that females have a higher prevalence of SAD than males, in contrast to older studies that found no gender differences. As with other anxiety disorders, SAD appears to aggregate in families.

Etiology

A variety of theoretical perspectives on the etiology of SAD exist. The high familial concurrence of anxiety disorders makes it difficult to separate the contributions of genetic inheritance, temperament, family dynamics, modeling, and other environmental factors. An interactive mechanism is most likely.

Developmental theorists focus on the interplay between the exploring toddler's normal uncertainty about the location of the caregiver and the at-risk child's anxious or insecure attachment. Behaviorally oriented theories emphasize the maintenance of symptoms by conditioned fear, based on stimulus generalization and reinforcement. Recent research using an attachment theory model found that insecure mother-infant attachment and maternal sensitivity each separately predicted separation anxiety in children at age 6 years (Dallaire and Weinraub 2005).

Biological theories focus on temperamental, genetic, and physiological factors. More specifically, research reveals age-specific effects of both genes and shared environment on anxiety, depression, and withdrawn behavior in childhood and adolescence (Lamb et al. 2010). Mood or anxiety disorders are commonly found in the parents and other relatives of children with SAD. A possible subtype of SAD has been identified in children who may be at particularly high risk for developing panic disorder as adults (Roberson-Nay et al. 2010). *Behavioral inhibition* as described by Kagan (1998) refers to a genetically based temperament trait whereby children respond to a new or unfamiliar situation with avoidance, distress, caution, and/or reticence. Both family studies of subjects with anxiety disorders and prospective studies of toddlers have found that behavioral inhibition is correlated with increased risk of developing anxiety disorders. Specific parenting styles characterized by rejection, control, and intrusiveness are also likely related to increased anxiety in youth (Muris et al. 1998; Rapee 1997; Wood 2006).

Course and Prognosis

SAD typically begins around school age and is usually recognized in early or middle childhood. The disorder is often recurrent, with acute exacerbations at the beginning of the school year, following holiday breaks from school, or when starting a new school. Precipitants include actual separations, parental divorce, deaths, family moves, family changes, or crises. Symptoms may worsen during or after medical illnesses or procedures. As in most childhood psychiatric disorders, comorbidity with other anxiety and non-anxiety disorders is common, although rates vary among studies.

Most children who suffer from SAD never receive mental health treatment. A substantial proportion of children with SAD eventually recover, with or without treatment. Others experience repeated remissions and relapses, and may develop a chronic course with impairment extending into adulthood. In addition to suggested links between childhood SAD and adult agoraphobia or panic disorder, SAD may be considered a general risk factor for depression and anxiety disorders.

Follow-up studies of childhood school absenteeism have reported a high prevalence of adult maladaptation and psychiatric symptoms. Although these children tend to return to school eventually, many have poor overall emotional and social functioning. Because children with excessive school absences are heterogeneous, they have a variety of symptoms. School absentees often have academic underachievement and social avoidance and can be at risk for excessive absenteeism from work or chronic unemployment in adulthood.

Evaluation and Differential Diagnosis

A parent may need to be present with the child for the entire initial interview, if separation is too difficult. Evaluation should include probing for symptoms of anxiety or mood disorders in both the child and the parents, assessing for syndromes that may mimic anxiety, and using rating scales to quantify symptoms whenever possible. Physical symptoms such as nausea, vomiting, abdominal pain, or headaches require judicious medical evaluation. In SAD, somatic symptoms are typically worse on evenings and mornings before school and absent on weekends and holidays, except as separations approach. Learning or language disorders should be ruled out. A careful focus is needed on identifying any factors contributing to school refusal, using multiple informants (child, parent, teacher, other school staff).

Separation anxiety is a normal developmental phenomenon at ages 6–30 months, with intensification between 13 and 18 months of age (Kearney et al. 2003). In children younger than 6 years, normal separation anxiety can reappear in stressful situations. In an older child, this may represent an *adjustment disorder with anxiety.* Other anxiety disorders in the differential diagnosis include *generalized anxiety disorder, panic disorder,* and *simple or social phobia.* A *depressive disorder* may also cause clinginess and refusal to separate from the parent. Children with *schizophrenia, autistic disorder,* or *pervasive developmental disorder not otherwise specified* may present with symptoms of separation anxiety.

When evaluating the patient with chronic school absenteeism, the clinician should investigate possible causes other than separation anxiety (see Table 4–2). The most common cause of school absenteeism in adolescents is truancy, a feature of *conduct disorder.* Youngsters with truancy typically show delinquent behavior. They may leave home in the morning and spend the day with friends, while their parents are unaware of or not concerned about their activities, in contrast to children with SAD, who remain at home with their parents' knowledge.

Treatment

Psychosocial Treatments

SAD is treated using a multimodal approach, including psycho-education, collaboration with primary care providers, school consultation, cognitive-behavioral therapy (CBT), family therapy, and selective serotonin reuptake inhibitors (SSRIs).

School absenteeism requires prompt intervention because, regardless of the cause, the longer the child is out of school, the higher the likelihood of treatment resistance, chronicity, and school failure. The goals are age-appropriate separation of parent and child and a rapid return to school. Referral to a partial hospitalization program (day treatment) (see Chapter 9) may be warranted as a transition to school reentry, particularly if school refusal persists despite adequate outpatient treatment. Treatment focuses on CBT, while enlisting the cooperation of the family and the school. As described by Kearney and Albano (2000), relaxation training, cognitive modification, social skills training, exposure-based activities, and contracting and contingency management are the key CBT components. Specific techniques include limit setting, eliminating secondary gain for staying home, escorts to school, gradual exposure to increasing lengths of time at school, and rewarding the child for increasing successful attendance. Proactive problem-solving around any school issues such as bullying is essential. Home schooling is contraindicated. Multimodal treatment planning for youth with SAD must be done sensitively, with understanding of the child's symptoms and concerns. If the child also has panic disorder or a major depressive episode, aggressive return to school prior to addressing these comorbid issues can exacerbate symptoms. A thoughtful treatment plan for school reentry includes planning calm and predictable morning routines, encouraging children and parents to use new cognitive-behavioral skills, addressing positive and/or negative reinforcement of school refusal behavior, and ensuring safety in the environment (such as a school social worker providing support during the school day). Classroom-based accommodations and modifications may also be appropriate under an Individualized Education Plan or Response to Intervention planning.

The psychotherapeutic treatment with the strongest empirical support for treatment of SAD in youth is CBT. This time-limited therapy focuses on psychoeducation of parents and youth, management of somatic symptoms, problem solving, cognitive restructuring, behavioral exposures, and relapse prevention (Velting et al. 2004). Parent-child interaction therapy (PCIT) may be an effective treatment for younger children, although research is limited. Given enhanced outcomes of combination treatment (sertraline plus CBT) compared with either treatment alone in a recent large study (Walkup et al. 2008), an SSRI plus CBT is most effective for youth with SAD, generalized anxiety disorder, and/or social phobia. However, depending on availability, cost, time factors, and family preference, any of these treatments (an SSRI, CBT, or combination treatment) may be selected in an individual case. Individual psychodynamic psychotherapy has been used and may help children with SAD to resolve conflicts and achieve improved self-esteem and mastery over separation and autonomy. This therapy actively involves parents as well. However, empirical support for this approach is very limited.

Common issues in any modality of SAD treatment are planned and unplanned absences (e.g., vacations by the patient or therapist, school transitions, parental absence, losses of people important to the child) and the termination of treatment. Anticipatory guidance for the parents and the child regarding expected separations is useful. Once treatment is completed, the therapist should be specific about when and how to return to treatment, for example at times of increased vulnerability or if symptoms return.

Pharmacotherapy

An antidepressant may be added to the treatment of separation anxiety or comorbid mood disorder when moderate to severe anxiety symptoms persist despite appropriate psychosocial and family-based therapeutic interventions. SSRIs have replaced imipramine and other tricyclic antidepressants (TCAs) as a result of their more favorable side-effect profile and improved tolerability. The age of the child should always be taken into consideration. Older children are more commonly treated with medication than younger children. Benzodiazepines have been used rarely as adjuncts to psychological interventions, although behavioral disinhibition, sedation, and dependence/withdrawal are serious potential side effects. These agents should be used sparingly, temporarily, and in combination with an SSRI, if at all.

Other Interventions

Firm limit setting is necessary in treating truancy. When school absenteeism includes family permission, socializing with peers, risk of physical danger, or substance abuse, appropriate social interventions and referrals/consultations are indicated.

SAD-related sleep disturbance or resistance to sleeping alone is generally treated behaviorally. Techniques include developing a predictable and calming bedtime routine, monitoring of bedtime behavior, teaching the child relaxation and other coping skills, and supporting parents while coaching them to positively reinforce the child for sleeping in his or her own bed (McMenamy and Katz 1989).

If a parent's own anxiety or mood disorder is making it harder to separate from the child, the parent should also receive direct psychiatric treatment (possibly including appropriate medication) in addition to guidance in child management and parenting in the context of individual or family therapy.

Severe SAD that results in total avoidance of school and does not respond to environmental, psychotherapeutic, and pharmacological interventions may require psychiatric hospitalization. However, prompt referral to a partial hospitalization program (day treatment) can often prevent the need for inpatient hospitalization. When available, intensive outpatient programs (IOP) that offer treatment several days a week (typically after school) can also be useful as a "step up" from traditional outpatient care if more intensive treatment is needed, or as a "step down" to ease the transition to school reentry following hospitalization or partial hospitalization.

■ FEEDING AND EATING DISORDERS OF INFANCY OR EARLY CHILDHOOD

Pica

Clinical Description

Pica, a pattern of eating nonfood materials, may occur in young children, mentally retarded individuals, chronically anxious persons, and pregnant women. It is culturally normative in certain regions of the world. Pica is minimally documented in the psychiatric literature, despite the presumed biopsychosocial etiology and major potential behavioral, cognitive, neurological, and developmental complications. Pica in children most often comes to clinical attention in association with other behavior and medical problems.

Epidemiology

Up to one-third of young children are believed to exhibit pica at some point in their lives. It may be normative in children younger than 3 years. Low socioeconomic status, environmental deprivation, and parental psychopathology appear to be risk factors. The prevalence of the problem in mentally retarded individuals increases with the severity of the retardation.

Etiology

Etiological possibilities include nutritional deficiencies, insufficient stimulation, parent–child relationship difficulties, or cultural tradition, although there is no definitive support for any of these.

Course and Prognosis

Pica usually starts at age 12–24 months and resolves by school age except in mentally retarded persons, who may have pica into adulthood. Common forms of pica include ice, lead, clay, or soil ingestion. Delayed motor and mental development, neurological deficits, and behavioral abnormalities may predate (and perhaps contribute to) or result from pica.

Pica has numerous potentially severe medical complications, including heavy metal poisoning, parasitic infections, or intestinal obstruction. Lead toxicity (from ingestion of peeling paint, dust from home renovation, plaster, or soil) can lead to learning disorders, hyperactivity, fatigue, weight loss, and constipation, and even to toxic encephalopathy.

Evaluation and Differential Diagnosis

Pica should be considered in all cases of developmental delays, learning difficulties, mental retardation, unusual behavioral symptoms, and chronic constipation. In order to diagnose pica, the clinician must do a behavioral and psychiatric evaluation of the child and parents, and determine the child's nutritional status and feeding history. Inadequate supervision of children or parental neglect should be considered. Questions should be asked about peeling paint or renovation in the home that might increase lead exposure.

Unexplained fatigue or weight loss, learning impairments, mental retardation, or gingival "lead lines" can be signs of lead poisoning; however, most children with elevated blood lead levels have no symptoms. Periodic blood tests for lead in children with pica are recommended. Consultation with pediatric colleagues is indicated if blood lead levels are elevated (>10 µg/dL).

Treatment

Behavior therapy has been successful in mentally retarded individuals with pica and may be applicable to other children. Components include education, the rewarding of appropriate eating, and teaching the differentiation of edible foods. Appropriate responses to instances of pica include overcorrection (enforced immediate oral hygiene) and negative reinforcement (time-outs, restriction of privileges), combined with a positive reinforcement contingency behavior plan (reward system). Additional interventions include increased supervision, promotion of appropriate stimulation, improvement of play opportunities, or placement in day care. Concomitant treatment of medical complications may be required.

Rumination Disorder of Infancy

Clinical Description

Rumination disorder of infancy is a rare but potentially fatal eating disorder. Ruminating infants regurgitate and rechew their food in the absence of an associated gastrointestinal illness or dysfunction. Rumination may start with the infant placing fingers or clothes in the mouth to induce vomiting, with rhythmic body or neck motions, or without any apparent initiating action. During rumination, the infant generally lies quietly and looks happy or "spacey"; the body and head may be held in a characteristic arching position while sucking. When not ruminating, the infant may appear apathetic and withdrawn, become irritable and fussy, or seem quite normal. Various self-stimulatory behaviors, such as thumb sucking, cloth sucking, head banging, and body rocking, are commonly seen in association with rumination disorder.

Etiology

The etiology is unknown. One study (Whelan and Cooper 2000) found a strong relationship between maternal eating disorders and childhood feeding problems, although it is unclear whether this is genetically and/or environmentally mediated. Rumination is highly associated with gastroesophageal reflux.

Clinicians generally presume that the infant, lacking external sources of gratification, uses rumination for self-stimulation or social reinforcement. Although an understimulating or overstimulating environment can contribute to the appearance of rumination disorder, some infants with the disorder appear happy and have emotionally supportive and interactive parents. Thus, this disorder is a heterogeneous one. Children with severe and persistent feeding problems tend to have mental retardation, physical disabilities, medical illnesses, or developmental delays.

Course and Prognosis

Rumination typically occurs during the first year of life. It usually resolves by the end of the second year but may persist for another year or two. Spontaneous remissions are common. Tooth decay, failure to thrive, dehydration, electrolyte imbalance, and malnutrition can be complications.

A complication is the parental reaction to the symptoms. A parent's typical immediate response to the observance of rumination is anxiety and distress, with ongoing reactions that may impair parental attachment to the child. The parents' frustration and disgust, particularly at the odor, may lead to avoidance and understimulation of the child.

Evaluation and Differential Diagnosis

Behavioral and psychiatric evaluation of the child and parents emphasizes developmental history and psychosocial assessment, feeding and eating history, nutritional status, attachment, and observation of parent–child interactions during feeding. Medical conditions must be considered. Usually, children with rumination disorder appear happy and enjoy the regurgitation, whereas children with gastrointestinal disorders vomit with discomfort and experience pain, but this distinction is often not clear in practice. The clinician should carefully evaluate esophageal and gastric function in conjunction with the psychiatric evaluation.

Treatment

Behavioral consultation is highly recommended in treating rumination disorder. Parent training focusing on behavioral techniques including positive attention and interaction (cuddling and playing with the child before, during, and after mealtimes) will reduce social deprivation and behavioral withdrawal. Negative attention, such as shouting or physical discipline, can actually reinforce the behavior, especially if other forms of reinforcement and attention are lacking or ineffective. Negative reinforcement (ignoring) combined with a reward for time not ruminating (parental attention and social interaction, such as playing) can be used in outpatient treatment.

Pediatric hospitalization may be necessary for severe cases of malnutrition. By providing a partial separation of the child from the primary caregiver, an alternative feeding environment for the child (to "decondition" the symptoms), and a period of respite for the parent, hospitalization can be effective. Reassurance, education, and support of the parents help to reduce their anxiety and avoidance and establish the parents' comfort in the feeding process. Continuing treatment facilitates attachment between infant and parent, monitors the psychosocial environment at home, and provides support in the event of emerging mental retardation or other developmental problems.

■ TOURETTE'S DISORDER AND OTHER TIC DISORDERS

Clinical Description

"A *tic* is a sudden, rapid, recurrent, nonrhythmic, stereotyped motor movement or vocalization" (American Psychiatric Association 2000, p. 100). Although tics are experienced as involuntary, they may be temporarily suppressed by conscious effort. They are often preceded by an "urge" to make a certain tic. DSM-IV-TR subdivides tic disorders into Tourette's disorder, chronic motor or vocal tic disorder, and transient tic disorder. Tourette's disorder is characterized by its chronicity and the presence at some time of both motor and vocal tics. Unlike other DSM-IV-TR disorders, functional impairment is not required to make the diagnosis (American Psychiatric Association 2000).

Epidemiology

Simple tics are extremely frequent, especially in school-age boys. Tourette's disorder is up to 3 times more prevalent in boys than girls. The prevalence of Tourette's disorder may be higher than traditionally thought, according to a population-based epidemiological study in 13- to 14-year-olds in mainstream schools that found a rate of 0.8%–1.8% (Hornsey et al. 2001). Milder forms of chronic tics are far more common than full Tourette's disorder.

Comorbidity

Comorbid disorders are common and are often more disabling than the tics. About one-half of children with Tourette's disorder referred to psychiatric clinics also have ADHD. Oppositional behavior is also common, and anger dyscontrol can impede functioning. Obsessive-compulsive symptoms are often present, with up to 60% of patients with Tourette's disorder meeting criteria for obsessive-compulsive disorder (OCD) at some time. OCD is typically associated with a more severe Tourette's presentation. Other anxiety disorders may correlate with tic severity in Tourette's disorder (Coffey et al. 2000). Depression is also prevalent in these patients.

Tourette's disorder and explosivity may represent a common comorbid presentation (Budman et al. 2000). Cohrs et al. (2001) observed markedly disturbed sleep in patients with Tourette's syndrome, which correlated with symptom severity during the day.

Etiology

Tourette's disorder is considered to be a neuropsychiatric illness with a variety of etiologies. There is increasing evidence suggesting cortical-striatal-thalamic circuit involvement. Numerous neurotransmitters have been implicated.

Extensive genetic research supports the high heritability of this disorder. The concordance rate in monozygotic twins is about 55%. The interactions of genetic and (biological) environmental influences are complex. Genetic linkage studies have not been conclusive, and the disorder appears to be genetically heterogeneous.

Pediatric autoimmune neuropsychiatric disorders associated with streptococcal group A β-hemolytic streptococcal infections

(PANDAS) are characterized by a relapsing-remitting symptom pattern with significant psychiatric comorbidity that may include affective, behavioral, anxiety, and cognitive symptoms. Some cases of Tourette's disorder (and of OCD), particularly those with sudden onset or exacerbation, have been linked to antineuronal antibodies resulting from group A β-hemolytic streptococcal infections. This association remains controversial.

Approximately 10% of children with ADHD have tics, regardless of treatment with stimulant medication. Stimulants and some antidepressants may temporarily aggravate tics, but they do not appear to cause tic disorders or hasten the appearance of tics in a vulnerable child. Medication use is often simply coincidental with the onset of tics, which naturally wax and wane.

Course and Prognosis

Symptoms of tic disorders typically wax and wane, and the location of tics changes over time. Transitions or stressors, such as the start of the school year, vacations, and family disruption or geographic move, typically precipitate increased frequency and severity of tics. Anxiety, pleasurable excitement, boredom, or fatigue can exacerbate tics.

Onset of Tourette's disorder is typically during childhood and early adolescence. Symptoms of ADHD often appear before any tics. Seven years is the mean age at onset of motor symptoms, which usually begin as a single motor tic and have a rostrocaudal (head before trunk and limbs) progression over time. Motor tics can include eye blinking, eyebrow raising, facial grimacing, head jerks, abdominal tics, and leg/foot movements. Complex gestures may appear later. Complex motor tics may appear purposeless or may be camouflaged by being blended into purposeful movements. They may mirror someone else's movements (echokinesis or echopraxia). By age 9–10 years, many patients with Tourette's disorder can describe premonitory sensory urges (uncomfortable feelings in a specific part of the body that are relieved with the performance of a tic).

At an average age of 11 years, phonic and vocal tics may appear, along with obsessions and compulsive behaviors. Vocal tics may start as a single syllable or sounds such as throat clearing, grunting, sniffing, snorting, or barking, and progress to longer exclamations. Classic coprolalia (swearing or obscene language) is present in fewer than 10% of patients with Tourette's disorder. Other complex vocal tics include palilalia (repeating one's own sounds) and echolalia (repeating others' words).

In most cases, the severity of symptoms diminishes after puberty; about one-third recover by late adolescence, and another one-third significantly improve by adulthood. In the remaining one-third, symptoms range from mild to (rarely) severe.

Complications of Tourette's disorder include self-consciousness, shame, impaired self-esteem and social adaptation, and avoidance of social situations that result from being teased and rejected by peers and even parents and teachers. Severe symptoms may interfere with forming satisfying friendships and romantic relationships. The unemployment rate in adults with Tourette's disorder is reportedly as high as 50%. Comorbid illnesses, including mood disorders, self-injurious behavior, or anxiety disorders, can also contribute to impairment.

Evaluation and Differential Diagnosis

Patients with Tourette's disorder often attempt to hide symptoms or are unaware of them. They typically suppress tics while in the physician's office. As a result, the physician may underestimate the severity or overlook the diagnosis altogether. There are often many years between the first symptoms and the diagnosis.

Neurological history and examination are needed to rule out other movement disorders. Baseline dyskinesias should be assessed before medication is started. If myoclonic seizures are suspected, an electroencephalogram may be helpful.

Psychiatric evaluation focuses on identifying concomitant anxiety, mood, behavior, and developmental disorders and stressors that may be exacerbating symptoms. Specific questions regarding obsessions and compulsions are indicated. School reports of academic performance, standardized test results, tic severity, social skills, and behavioral observations are useful. If school performance is impaired, psychological testing that includes assessment of intellectual functioning and academic achievement can clarify the diagnosis of a comorbid learning disorder or lower intellectual capacity. Other possible interference with school success includes direct effects of tics or premonitory urges, efforts to suppress tics or compulsions, intrusive obsessions, ADHD, anxiety symptoms, social stigmatization, cognitive dulling or anxiety secondary to medication, and excessive absenteeism. The clinician evaluates the child's self-consciousness, ability to manage peer teasing, social ostracism, and assertiveness. Family history of tics and associated disorders is important, and evaluation of relatives for tic disorders may be considered.

The differential diagnosis includes a wide variety of *neurological disorders* that present with involuntary movements. Patients with *autistic disorder* or *stereotypic movement disorder* may have stereotyped movements that resemble tics. *Normal* children may have isolated, fleeting tics, but such twitches (blinks, grimaces) and habits are not diagnosed even as a transient tic disorder unless they persist nearly every day for at least 4 weeks. The clinical boundaries between Tourette's disorder, *ADHD,* and *OCD* are blurred in many patients who have symptoms of all three disorders. Complex tics may be difficult to distinguish from compulsions, and some patients have both.

Treatment

Transient tics do not require treatment. The clinician should advise the family to reduce attention to the symptom and avoid criticism. The clinician may also educate and reassure the patient and family and encourage them to return if symptoms persist. Chronic tic disorder alone rarely requires specific treatment unless the tics are disabling, in which case the same treatments may be used as for Tourette's disorder (see below). There is evidence that tics are highly associated with school problems; therefore, special education programming may be indicated (Kurlan et al. 2001).

For Tourette's disorder, a period of initial monitoring helps to establish a baseline of symptom severity. A log or diary can be useful. Children are often brought to clinical attention at a time of crisis, and the evaluation itself, along with reassurance about the nature of the illness, may result in a decrease in symptoms and distress.

Psychosocial Treatments

Education of the patient and parents, teachers, and peers ameliorates the social consequences of tics. Referral to the Tourette Syndrome Association (local chapter and/or Web site; www.tsa-usa.org) may be invaluable to provide information and support. Psychosocial interventions often precede pharmacological treatment. In many cases, the control of tics is less urgent than the treatment of the accompanying attentional, behavioral, or obsessive-compulsive symptoms. A recent controlled study demonstrated the efficacy of a comprehensive behavioral intervention including habit reversal (a competing response procedure) (Piacentini et al. 2010). Supportive psychotherapy may help an individual cope with the stigma of illness, promote self-esteem, improve interpersonal comfort and social skills, and improve anxiety. Family therapy may assist in reducing the child's stress and helping the family manage associated symptoms. Behavior modification at home and school is recommended for comorbid symptoms of ADHD and ODD. CBT may be used for obsessive-compulsive symptoms. A school Individualized Education Program (IEP) with tutoring, resource room, or special education classroom may be indicated for children with comorbid learning disabilities or behavior problems.

Pharmacotherapy

Medication treatment is complicated by possible side effects and the difficulty in determining effectiveness because of the disorder's natural waxing and waning course. The goal is not to eliminate tics but to reduce them to a level that does not interfere with the child's development and functioning. The first step in pharmacologic treatment planning is to identify the most troubling target symptoms and choose a medication that is likely to address those symptoms while producing the fewest side effects.

In a randomized controlled trial in children with comorbid tics and ADHD, guanfacine improved teacher and clinician ratings (but not parent ratings) of ADHD symptoms, decreased errors on a continuous performance test (subjects on placebo had increased errors), and decreased tic severity (Scahill et al. 2001). Treatment of tics with clonidine has some empirical support and may also improve sleep and symptoms of ADHD. Guanfacine is associated with less sedation and vital sign changes than is clonidine. Both drugs now have long-acting forms.

The use of stimulants to treat symptoms of ADHD in the presence of tics has been controversial. Current practice is to balance the possible risk of tic exacerbation with the impairment caused by the ADHD symptoms. Although stimulants are safe and effective for many children with tics, careful monitoring is prudent to evaluate for possible stimulant-induced tic exacerbation. A recent multisite randomized controlled trial found that methylphenidate and clonidine (particularly in combination) were effective for ADHD in children with accompanying tics (Tourette's Syndrome Study Group 2002). Mean tic severity improved in all three active treatment conditions, but most with combination treatment. Clonidine was most helpful for impulsivity and hyperactivity; methylphenidate was most helpful for inattention. The proportion of subjects whose tics worsened was no higher in those treated with methylphenidate (20%) than in those on clonidine alone (26%) or placebo (22%). Clonidine commonly caused sedation, but there was no evidence of cardiac toxicity, whether used alone or combined with methylphenidate. Amphetamine may be more prone to increase tics than methylphenidate is. Atomoxetine is an alternative medication for symptoms of ADHD and has not been observed to increase tics.

For severe tics, an atypical antipsychotic or the older neuroleptic drug pimozide can be used, but all have problematic side effects. SSRIs are effective for OCD symptoms but not for tic reduction.

■ ELIMINATION DISORDERS

Encopresis

Clinical Description

Encopresis is defined as fecal soiling of clothes or excretion in inappropriate places that occurs at least once a month for at least 3 months. The child's chronological and developmental age must be at least 4 years, when full bowel control is developmentally expected. Medical evaluation is necessary before labeling the disorder as "functional."

Encopresis typically occurs during the day. Many children deny the problem even when the odor is obvious or stool is discovered in their underwear. In half of these patients, bowel control is not yet learned, so the encopresis is termed *primary*. In *secondary* encopresis, the child learned bowel control, was continent for at least 1 year, and then regressed. Between 50% and 60% of encopretic children have secondary encopresis. Boys with primary encopresis are more likely than those with the secondary form to also have developmental delay and enuresis.

Children may have constipation or voluntary stool withholding with continuous leaking overflow incontinence, a problem that resolves with treatment of the constipation. This problem is classified as "retentive encopresis." Children with incontinence without constipation, or "nonretentive encopresis," tend to produce formed stools that they may leave for discovery.

Epidemiology

Prevalence of encopresis gradually decreases with age and is reported in approximately 3% of 4-year-olds, 2% of 6-year-olds, and 1.6% of 10- to 11-year-olds. The problem is rare in adolescents. Among school-age children, males predominate in ratios from 2.5:1 to 6:1. Higher rates are observed among individuals with mental retardation.

Etiology

Retentive encopresis may initially be triggered by painful defecation, inadequate or punitive toilet training, fear of using the school bathroom, or toilet-related fears. Once retention and constipation are initiated by emotional or medical factors, bowel physiology may maintain them independently. Parents may not recognize that the soiling is related to chronic constipation rather than reluctance to use the toilet. Pathophysiological mechanisms include altered colon motility and contraction patterns, obstruction, stretched and thinned colon walls (megacolon), and decreased sensation or perception secondary to a neurological disorder. Liquid stool leaks around the impaction, and the child is unaware and unable to exert control. Studies that examine the physiological causes of encopresis do not clearly differentiate between problems caused by primary organic pathology and those due to emotionally initiated chronic constipation.

Encopresis may result from stress-induced diarrhea, a problem related to irritable bowel syndrome in adulthood. Nonretentive encopresis may be a deliberate attempt by the child to effect change, as a means of avoiding stressors or communicating anger. These cases are typically more complicated and difficult to treat.

Course and Prognosis

Secondary encopresis usually starts by age 8 years. Among patients who have constipation and encopresis before age 4 years, 63% recover with treatment. Of children older than 5 years who were placed on a laxative protocol in an encopresis clinic, 50% were able to discontinue the laxatives with no symptom recurrence after 1 year; another 20% discontinued the laxatives after 2 years (Loening-Baucke 1989). Psychiatric or medical comorbidity may be the primary determinant of prognosis.

Behavior problems are more common in the psychiatrically referred population than in those seen by pediatricians. In the psychiatric population, 25% of children with encopresis also have enuresis. In the pediatric population, patients will occasionally suffer from a symptom complex that includes urinary tract infection, encopresis, and constipation. Treatment of the constipation and urinary tract infection may resolve all of the symptoms, without a need for urologic examination. Some children withhold both urine and feces and may have megabladder and megacolon.

Evaluation and Differential Diagnosis

A detailed history of bowel function, nature and pattern of soiling, attempts to train or treat, and bathroom habits and environment is needed. Physical examination should include an abdominal examination for evidence of a fecal mass, an anal examination for evidence of fecal material, a rectal digital examination for stool consistency, and a neurological examination with perianal sensation testing. The need for additional laboratory tests is based on the history and physical examination. A barium enema is not necessary in uncomplicated cases of encopresis but may be helpful in diagnosing *Hirschsprung's disease* (congenital megacolon). Urinalysis will detect a secondary urinary tract infection, which is common in girls with encopresis. *Medical causes of fecal incontinence* include thyroid disease, hypercalcemia, lactase deficiency, pseudo-obstruction, myelomeningocele (spina bifida), cerebral palsy with hypotonia, rectal stenosis, anal fissure, Hirschsprung's disease (which is usually associated, however, with large feces rather than incontinence), and anorectal trauma.

Psychiatric evaluation includes assessment for associated psychiatric disorders. Oppositional children may soil willfully. Children with ADHD do not plan ahead, so they may be caught by an urge to defecate when a bathroom is not available. They also may be prone to constipation (because of spending insufficient time toileting) or fecal soiling of underwear (due to careless hygiene). Anxious children may be intimidated by perceived or real dangers or humiliations in school bathrooms and avoid defecation, only to have an "accident" on the way home.

Treatment

Most cases of encopresis can be treated by a pediatrician, but more complex cases need psychological intervention. The pediatrician educates the child and parents about bowel function. For encopresis without constipation, a behavior shaping program gives rewards first for just sitting on the toilet and later for moving the bowels appropriately. A negative consequence for soiling may be used. Manipulative soiling requires parent management training and a reduction of reinforcers for maladaptive behavior. For children with severe stool retention, impaction, and loss of bowel tone, initial bowel cleaning (e.g., with enemas or suppositories) followed by "retraining" the bowel (e.g., with stool softener or mineral oil, a high-fiber diet, development of a toileting routine, and use of a mild suppository if necessary) may be used in conjunction with the behavioral program. Repeated administration of enemas by parents is harmful to the parent–child relationship. Benefit is possible from the adjunctive use of hypnosis or biofeedback to improve sphincter control, although solid empirical evidence is lacking. Individual and family psychiatric interventions are indicated in resistant cases, in which the focus of treatment shifts to the associated psychiatric disorders. The role of psychopharmacology in the treatment of these children is relatively insignificant.

Enuresis

Clinical Description

Urinary incontinence in young children, and occasionally in older children after toilet training has been completed, may be a normal developmental phenomenon. The mechanisms involved in learning bladder control are not well understood. *Enuresis* is diagnosed when wetting occurs after the chronological or developmental age of 5 years either at least twice a week for 3 months or sufficiently often to cause distress or impairment. The addition of subjective criteria allows the clinician to make the diagnosis in children who do not meet either the frequency or the duration criterion, but in whom wetting is accompanied by emotional upset or social consequences.

Bed wetting is more common than daytime incontinence. Nocturnal enuresis typically occurs 30 minutes to 3 hours after sleep onset but may occur at any time during the night. The child may sleep through the episode or be awakened by the moisture. Daytime bladder control usually precedes nocturnal control by 1–2 years. Most children with daytime enuresis also have nocturnal enuresis. Some clinicians do not diagnose nocturnal enuresis until the child is age 6 or 7 years. If bladder control has not yet been achieved, the enuresis is *primary*. In *secondary* enuresis, wetting reappears after a period of established urinary continence.

Epidemiology

Enuresis is seen in 5%–10% of 5-year-olds and around 3%–5% of 10-year-olds (American Psychiatric Association 2000). The male predominance of primary enuresis decreases with age. After age 5 years, the prevalence of enuresis in both boys and girls spontaneously decreases by 5%–10% per year. Between 3% and 9% of school-age girls experience daytime wetting (Mattsson and Gladh 2003). The general prevalence in older adolescents and adults is 1%. Few of the children with nocturnal enuresis also have diurnal enuresis or encopresis. In contrast, 50%–60% of patients with diurnal enuresis are likely to experience nocturnal incontinence. Enuresis is of the primary type in more than 85% of cases, a percentage that gradually decreases with age. Secondary enuresis is equally prevalent in boys and girls.

Etiology

Approximately 70% of children with enuresis (particularly boys) have a first-degree relative with enuresis. Studies of monozygotic and dizygotic twins show a strong genetic factor, although the mode of transmission is unclear. A "maturational" etiology is suggested in patients with primary enuresis who have small-volume voidings, short stature, low mean bone age, and delayed sexual maturation. Some patients have a relative inability to concentrate urine. In these cases the spontaneous remission rate is 15% per year (Forsythe and Redmond 1974). Research has not established that children suffering from enuresis have a smaller than average bladder capacity. Excessive fluid intake may contribute to the problem. Anatomical abnormalities of the urinary tract are not typical causes of enuresis and rarely warrant surgical interventions. Common physiological causes of diurnal enuresis in girls are vaginal reflux of urine, "giggle incontinence," and urgency incontinence. Enuresis is more common in patients with sleep disorders. Enuresis may be a side effect of certain medications.

Children experiencing enuresis are often emotionally upset, but the relationship between psychiatric disorder and enuresis is nonspecific, and causality has not been demonstrated. Anxious children may experience urinary frequency, resulting in daytime incontinence if toilet facilities are not readily available or if the child is fearful of certain bathrooms. In ODD, refusal to use the toilet may be part of the child's battle for control. Children with either primary or secondary enuresis are more likely to meet diagnostic criteria for ADHD, although the etiologic connection is unproven. However, many children with ADHD wait until the last minute to urinate and then lose control on the way to the bathroom. Secondary enuresis may be related to stress, trauma, or psychosocial crisis. Enuresis that continues into adolescence is associated with higher rates of psychopathology.

Course and Prognosis

Primary enuresis has a high rate of spontaneous remission. Only about 1% of boys (and fewer girls) still have this condition at age 18 years. Secondary enuresis usually begins between ages 5 and 8 years. Onset in adolescence may signify more psychiatric problems and less favorable outcome.

Complications include embarrassment, anger from and punishment by caregivers, teasing by peers, avoidance of overnight visits and camp, social withdrawal, and angry outbursts. The development of psychiatric disorders is higher in enuretic children than in the general population.

Evaluation and Differential Diagnosis

Initial medical evaluation is required to rule out medical causes (Table 4–3), especially in secondary and diurnal enuresis. This in-

TABLE 4–3.	**Medical causes of urinary incontinence**

Urinary tract infection
Urethritis—bubble bath, sexual abuse
Diabetes mellitus
Diabetes insipidus
Sickle cell trait
Seizure disorder
Sleep apnea
Neurogenic bladder—myelodysplasia, trauma, other neurological disorder
Congenital malformation of the genitourinary tract
Urinary obstruction—stone, pelvic mass
Medication side effect

cludes a medical history (including questions about polyuria, dribbling, and urgency), a physical examination, observation of the size and velocity of the urine stream, and a urine culture and urinalysis. The osmolality result can help rule out diabetes mellitus or diabetes insipidus. In the absence of suggestive findings on the history and physical examination, invasive evaluation of the urinary tract is not indicated. Enuresis during both day and night and difficulty with voiding are indications of urinary tract abnormalities that may warrant investigation. A family history of diabetes or renal disease may suggest additional testing. A family history of enuresis is generally reassuring and implies that it will eventually be outgrown.

Psychiatric evaluation of the child and family includes assessment of associated psychiatric symptoms, recent psychosocial stressors, and family concern about and management of the symptoms. Developmental evaluation can identify the child who is not mature enough to achieve continence.

Treatment

Many cases of enuresis can be managed successfully by the pediatrician. For younger children who wet only at night, the most useful strategy is to minimize symptoms by advising the parents not to punish or ridicule the child while awaiting maturation. Children can be taught to change their own beds to reduce negative parental reactions. Restricting fluids before bedtime and waking the child after 2–3 hours of sleep to urinate are only occasionally useful.

For older children who are motivated to stop bed wetting, a monitoring and reward procedure (a chart with stars to be exchanged for rewards) may be effective. Daytime urinary continence may be achieved rapidly with a behavioral program. A program of "bladder training" exercises may be helpful. Practice in delaying bladder emptying may increase bladder capacity. Interruption of the stream while urinating may strengthen sphincter muscles and improve awareness of bladder sensations. Instruction on adapted voiding posture and hygiene may be effective for urethrovaginal reflux (Mattsson and Gladh 2003).

If simple interventions are unsuccessful, a urine alarm is recommended. This device, an improvement on the "bell and pad," has a high success rate of 75% at 6 months and 56% at 12 months. This compares favorably to rates of 6% at 6 months and 16% at 12 months using observation alone. If the alarm is set up to awaken the parents so they awaken the child, the relapse rate is low. A combination of the urine alarm, cleanliness training, retention control, and overlearning can stop bed wetting in two-thirds of children with primary enuresis (Houts et al. 1983). (See Bennett 2005 in "Additional Reading.")

Although behavioral treatments consistently demonstrate higher success rates than medication, DDAVP (desmopressin) or low doses of imipramine at bedtime can be helpful in the short term in patients who are resistant to behavioral interventions, who need a rapid result (e.g., for camp), or who have daytime as well as nighttime enuresis. The majority of patients relapse when either type of medication is withdrawn (unless maturation has intervened). DDAVP is available in both a nasal spray and a newer oral form. It has a more benign side-effect profile than imipramine.

Psychotherapy is rarely useful in the treatment of enuresis. However, it may be indicated for the treatment of psychosocial sequelae of enuresis. Children who experience enuresis as a consequence of trauma or stress may also benefit from psychotherapeutic interventions. Associated disorders may require psychiatric treatment.

■ SELECTIVE MUTISM

Clinical Description

Children with selective mutism do not speak in one or several important settings despite having the ability to comprehend spoken language and to speak in other situations. Symptoms persist for at least 1 month and are severe enough to affect educational and interpersonal functioning. These children have an adequate knowledge of the language yet may experience specific developmental communication disorders. Typically, speech is normal at home when the child is alone with parents and siblings, but partial or total muteness appears in the presence of teachers, peers, and strangers or selectively in unfamiliar places or particular social situations. When these children are separated from a familiar or comfortable setting, they might use gestures, nods, monosyllabic responses, written notes, or whispers but avoid full vocalization. Many of these children are shy, anxious, withdrawn, socially inhibited, fearful of new experiences, and resistant to separation from parents. Some have oppositional behavior, as well.

Epidemiology

Selective mutism is estimated to occur in fewer than 1% of school-age children and typically begins between 3 and 8 years of age. Prevalence ranges from 0.3% to 0.8%, depending on the age of the population studied and the length of their exposure to school. Increased prevalence in immigrant families is reported.

Etiology

Explanations for the development of selective mutism vary widely. Emotional and physical trauma, such as witnessing or being victimized by physical or sexual abuse, are rarely a primary precipitant. Biological factors, including temperament and anxiety disorders, are more important contributors to etiology. Early hospitalization or family instability characterized by divorce, death, or frequent moves could contribute to the development of these symptoms.

There may be a link between selective mutism in children and social phobia in adults. These adults recall feeling intensely anxious as children when they were asked to speak, with accompanying symptoms that approximate panic. Selective mutism may have been an early observable form of developing social phobia. Parents of selectively mute children tend to have a variety of anxiety disorders including panic, separation anxiety, and social/performance anxiety.

Selectively mute children typically also experience developmental delays in speech and language. Approximately 25% of children with selective mutism also had delayed onset of speech, and 50% have a speech disorder or speech immaturities. The prevalence of mental retardation and neurological disorders is increased. These associations suggest a neurodevelopmental etiology or that developmental disorders may worsen communication impairments. Global mutism can result from cerebellar lesions and is known to accompany cerebellar hemorrhages, subarachnoid hemorrhages, vertebral artery injuries, basilar artery occlusion, and head trauma.

Course and Prognosis

The disorder is usually discovered when the child attends kindergarten or first grade and is expected to speak. Excessive shyness may be identified retrospectively. The diagnosis is typically made between 3 and 8 years of age. Symptoms may last for weeks, months, or years and usually resolve by age 10. When selective mutism persists beyond age 12, patients are less likely to completely recover. Complications of selective mutism include academic underachievement and impaired peer relationships. The child's persistent silence may lead to unhelpful special class and school placements. Many of these children have comorbid psychiatric problems, including social phobia, OCD, or school avoidance. In clinically referred samples, some patients have comorbid ODD. Social phobia may emerge in adulthood.

Evaluation and Differential Diagnosis

Standard psychiatric evaluation is indicated, including family history of language or anxiety disorders. Speech and language evaluation is warranted. The clinician should review the child's medical history for evidence of neurological injury or delay or hearing deficit, with neurological evaluation or audiological testing if indicated. Although the child may not speak directly to the clinician, observation of the quality of interaction and ability to communicate nonverbally can yield valuable information. The clinician should evaluate the possible presence of physical or sexual abuse, depression, and anxiety disorders.

The differential diagnosis of failure to speak includes *hearing impairment, mental retardation, communication disorder, aphasia, pervasive developmental disorders, schizophrenia,* and *conversion disorder.* Global impairment of speech is characteristic of all but the latter three disorders.

Treatment

First-line treatment is behavioral, combining office-based desensitization with active involvement of parents at home and teachers at school (Cohan et al. 2006). Speech and language therapy is often needed, as well. Therapy is based on the assumption that the child will speak again. Any form of communication is encouraged through behavioral plans that shape behavior by reinforcing attempts to speak. Short-term therapy may be effective, although more resistant cases may require longer-term treatment. Family therapy may help to identify and change dysfunctional patterns that maintain symptoms. Although teachers and parents often make accommodations to the child's muteness, it is better to maintain a clear expectation that the child talk and communicate, at least for a structured period of each session. The parents should be explicit with the child about these expectations: to talk at school and in therapy.

In cases resistant to psychosocial approaches, there is some evidence to support pharmacologic treatment with fluoxetine or sertraline.

■ REACTIVE ATTACHMENT DISORDER OF INFANCY OR EARLY CHILDHOOD

Clinical Description

Reactive attachment disorder of infancy or early childhood (RAD) is characterized by an inability to form normal interpersonal relationships and a persistent disturbance in the child's responsiveness in all social situations. The disorder appears before age 5 years and is preceded by a history of maltreatment, deprivation, or repeated changes in primary caregiver. The *inhibited type* includes children with inhibited, hypervigilant, or contradictory behaviors. Their responses to caregivers include a mixture of approach, avoidance, resistance to comforting, and frozen watchfulness. The *disinhibited type* is characterized by excessive and indiscriminate sociability with relative strangers and lack of selectivity in attachment figures. These children may lack empathy and show limited eye contact, poor impulse control, lack of conscience, and abnormal speech patterns.

The clinical presentation changes with age. In early infancy, diagnosis is based on the failure to achieve social developmental expectations: lack of eye tracking or responsive smiling by age 2 months, failure to play simple games or to reach out to be picked up by age 5 months, or failure to show overt behavioral signs of attachment and bonding to a parent by age 8 months. Infants appear lethargic, have a weak cry, show little body movement or activity, have excessive or disrupted sleep, gain weight slowly, and resist being held. There may be associated feeding disorders.

In childhood, odd social responses, weak interpersonal attachment, inappropriate excitability, and mood abnormalities are seen. The children may appear withdrawn, passive, and not interested in people (inhibited type) or, in the disinhibited type, may display overly rapid familiarity, inappropriate touching and clinging, and immediate emotional involvement that seems odd or unusual.

Epidemiology

RAD is considered to be extremely rare, although there are no good studies of prevalence. Suggestions of increasing prevalence may reflect changes in reporting of neglect and abuse or increased awareness of the diagnosis.

Etiology

By (DSM-IV-TR) definition, RAD requires evidence of pathogenic care. This can take the form of abuse, neglect, or impaired parenting. The majority of research has focused on young children reared in institutions. Frequent changes in the primary caregiver with a resulting inability of the child to form stable attachments are presumed to contribute to the disorder. Parents or caregivers may have major depression, psychosis, substance abuse, or mental retardation. They may be poor, uneducated, or isolated from social and emotional supports. They may be hostile or indifferent to the child or simply have insufficient skills, supports, and frustration tolerance to deal with a "difficult" child. RAD is not inevitable in the presence of abuse, neglect, and inadequate parenting. Other disorders may result (e.g., PTSD), or resilient children who are placed in nurturing environments can eventually develop normal attachments and social relationships.

Course and Prognosis

The prognosis of RAD varies from spontaneous remission to malnutrition, infection, and death. Nutritional or psychosocial deprivation may result in long-term behavior changes, short stature, and lowered intelligence quotient (IQ). If emotional deprivation continues but food intake is adequate, children may have improved body growth but show emotional problems and developmental delays.

Evaluation

RAD is diagnosed by observation of parent–child interactions and a decrease in the child's symptoms in response to adequate emotional and physical care. The clinical observer assesses physical and emotional nurturance, including the adult's capacity for empathy, appropriateness of level and timing of stimulation, attentiveness to the child's behavior, matching of expectations with the child's developmental level, and emotional reactions (e.g., anxiety, anger, indifference) to the child. A home visit may be indicated to evaluate the adequacy of housing, safety, and nutrition. Psychiatric evaluation of the parents is essential. Physical or sexual abuse or neglect may not be quickly or easily identifiable.

A medical examination is required to rule out chronic physical illness or disability that may be causing organic failure to thrive and to diagnose associated medical conditions that require treatment.

Pediatric hospitalization of infants or very young children helps to make the diagnosis. Removal from the home environment may permit normal feeding and sleeping patterns to be reestablished and parental caregiving capacity to be evaluated and remediated. It has not been demonstrated that RAD can be reliably diagnosed in older children.

Differential Diagnosis

Reactive attachment disorder can be differentiated from *pervasive developmental disorders* (including *autistic disorder*) by the improvement in cognitive and social deficits in a caring environment and the absence of abnormalities in speech, language, and social communication characteristic of PDD. *Depression* and *PTSD* are alternative psychiatric disorders to consider for the inhibited type. Some of the behaviors in the disinhibited type may resemble *ADHD*.

Treatment

Basic medical care, provision of adequate nurturance, and education and psychiatric treatment of parents are needed. Legal intervention may be indicated. If parents are unavailable or unable to improve the quality of care, placement in therapeutic foster care may be indicated. Hospitalization is often justified by the complexity of medical and psychiatric interventions. Outpatient therapy is recommended when the parent understands the nature and consequences of the disorder and actively and reliably participates in the treatment program. Parents may require a great deal of practical assistance in establishing a nurturing environment. Therapy with parent and child together provides opportunities to educate the parent and to model more nurturing behavior.

■ REFERENCES

American Psychiatric Association: Diagnostic and Statistical Manual of Mental Disorders, 4th Edition, Text Revision. Washington, DC, American Psychiatric Association, 2000

Bernstein GA, Rapoport JL, Leonard HL: Separation anxiety and generalized anxiety disorders, in Textbook of Child and Adolescent Psychiatry, 2nd Edition. Edited by Wiener JM. Washington, DC, American Psychiatric Press, 1996, pp 471–485

Black B: Separation anxiety disorder and panic disorder, in Anxiety Disorders in Children and Adolescents. Edited by March JS. New York, Guilford, 1995, pp 212–234

Breton JJ, Bereron L, Valla JP, et al: Quebec Child Mental Health Survey: prevalence of DSM-III-R mental health disorders. J Child Psychol Psychiatry 40:375–384, 1999

Budman CL, Bruun RD, Park KS, et al: Explosive outbursts in children with Tourette's disorder. J Am Acad Child Adolesc Psychiatry 39:1270–1276, 2000

Coffey BJ, Biederman J, Smoller JW, et al: Anxiety disorders and tic severity in juveniles with Tourette's disorder. J Am Acad Child Adolesc Psychiatry 39:562–568, 2000

Cohan LS, Chavira DA, Stein MB: Practitioner review: psychosocial interventions for children with selective mutism: a critical evaluation of the literature from 1990–2005. J Child Psychol Psychiatry 47:1085–1097, 2006

Cohrs S, Rasch T, Altmeyer S, et al: Decreased sleep quality and increased sleep related movements in patients with Tourette's syndrome. J Neurol Neurosurg Psychiatry 70:192–197, 2001

Dallaire DH, Weinraub M: Predicting children's separation anxiety at age 6: the contributions of infant-mother attachment security, maternal sensitivity, and maternal separation anxiety. Attach Hum Dev 7:393–408, 2005

Forsythe WI, Redmond A: Enuresis and spontaneous cure rate: study of 1129 enuretics. Arch Dis Child 49:259–263, 1974

Hornsey H, Banerjee S, Zeitlin H, et al: The prevalence of Tourette syndrome in 13–14-year-olds in mainstream school. J Child Psychol Psychiatry 42:1035–1039, 2001

Houts AC, Liebert RM, Padawer W: A delivery system for the treatment of primary enuresis. J Abnorm Child Psychol 11:513–520, 1983

Kagan J: Galen's Prophecy: Temperament in Human Nature. Boulder, CO, Westview Press, 1998

Kashani JH, Orvaschel H: A community study of anxiety in children and adolescents. Am J Psychiatry 147:313–318, 1990

Kearney CA, Albano AM: When Children Refuse School: A Cognitive-Behavioral Therapy Approach (Therapist Guide). San Antonio, TX, Psychological Corporation, 2000

Kearney CA, Sims KE, Pursell CR, et al: Separation anxiety disorder in young children: a longitudinal and family analysis. J Clin Child Adolesc Psychol 32:593–598, 2003

Kurlan R, McDermott MP, Deeley C, et al: Prevalence of tics in school children and association with placement in special education. Neurology 57:1383–1388, 2001

Lamb DJ, Middeldorp CV, van Beijsterveldt CE, et al: Heritability of anxious-depressive and withdrawn behavior: age-related changes during adolescence. J Am Acad Child Adolesc Psychiatry 49:248–255, 2010

Last CG, Francis G, Hersen M, et al: Separation anxiety and school phobia: a comparison using DSM-III criteria. Am J Psychiatry 144:653–657, 1987

Loening-Baucke V: Factors determining outcome in children with chronic constipation and faecal soiling. Gut 30:999–1006, 1989

Mattsson S, Gladh G: Urethrovaginal reflux: a common cause of daytime incontinence in girls. Pediatrics 111:136–139, 2003

McMenamy C, Katz RC: Brief parent-assisted treatment for children's nighttime fears. J Dev Behav Pediatr 10:145–148, 1989

Muris P, Meesters C, Merckelbach H, et al: Worry in normal children. J Am Acad Child Adolesc Psychiatry 37:703–710, 1998

Piacentini J, Woods DW, Scahill L, et al: Behavior therapy for children with Tourette disorder: a randomized controlled trial. JAMA 303:1929–1937, 2010

Rapee RM: Potential role of childrearing practices in the development of anxiety and depression. Clin Psychol Rev 17:47–67, 1997

Roberson-Nay R, Klein DF, Klein RG, et al: Carbon dioxide hypersensitivity in separation-anxious offspring of parents with panic disorder. Biol Psychiatry 67:1171–1177, 2010

Scahill L, Chappell P, Kim YS, et al: A placebo-controlled study of guanfacine in the treatment of children with tic disorders and attention deficit hyperactivity disorder. Am J Psychiatry 158:1067–1074, 2001

Shear K, Jin R, Ruscio AM, et al: Prevalence and correlates of estimated DSM-IV child and adult separation anxiety disorder in the National Comorbidity Survey Replication. Am J Psychiatry 163:1074–1083, 2006

Tourette's Syndrome Study Group: Treatment of ADHD in children with tics: a randomized controlled trial. Neurology 58:527–536, 2002

Velting ON, Setzer NJ, Albano AM: Update on and advances in assessment and cognitive-behavioral treatment of anxiety disorders in children and adolescents. Prof Psychol Res Pr 35:42–54, 2004

Walkup JT, Albano AM, Piacentini J, et al: Cognitive behavioral therapy, sertraline, or a combination in childhood anxiety. N Engl J Med 359:2753–2766, 2008

Whelan E, Cooper PJ: The association between childhood feeding problems and maternal eating disorder: a community study. Psychological Medicine 30:69–77, 2000

Wood JJ: Parental intrusiveness and children's separation anxiety in a clinical sample. Child Psychiatry Hum Dev 37:73–87, 2006

■ ADDITIONAL READING

Separation Anxiety Disorder

American Academy of Child and Adolescent Psychiatry: Practice parameter for the assessment and treatment of children and adolescents with anxiety disorders. J Am Acad Child Adolesc Psychiatry 46:267–283, 2007

Bernstein GA, Victor AM: Separation anxiety disorders and school refusal, in Dulcan's Textbook of Child and Adolescent Psychiatry. Edited by Dulcan MK. Washington, DC, American Psychiatric Publishing, 2010, pp 332–333

Tourette's Disorder and Other Tic Disorders

Towbin KE: Tic disorders, in Dulcan's Textbook of Child and Adolescent Psychiatry. Edited by Dulcan MK. Washington, DC, American Psychiatric Publishing, 2010, pp 417–434

Elimination Disorders

Bennett HJ: Waking Up Dry: A Guide to Help Children Overcome Bedwetting. Elk Grove Village, IL, American Academy of Pediatrics, 2005

Mikkelsen EJ: Elimination disorders, in Dulcan's Textbook of Child and Adolescent Psychiatry. Edited by Dulcan MK. Washington, DC, American Psychiatric Publishing, 2010, pp 435–448

Selective Mutism

Sharkey L, McNicholas F: 'More than 100 years of silence,' elective mutism: a review of the literature. Eur Child Adolesc Psychiatry 17:255–263, 2008

Reactive Attachment Disorder

American Academy of Child and Adolescent Psychiatry: Practice parameter for the assessment and treatment of children and adolescents with reactive attachment disorder of infancy and early childhood. J Am Acad Child Adolesc Psychiatry 44:1206–1219, 2005

5

"ADULT" DISORDERS THAT MAY BEGIN IN CHILDHOOD OR ADOLESCENCE

The disorders covered in this chapter are described in the general sections of DSM-IV-TR (American Psychiatric Association 2000), Axis I. Eating disorders may begin in adolescence (and, very rarely, prior to puberty), but bulimia typically begins in young adulthood. Substance-related disorders and schizophrenia have a similar pattern of peak incidence in early adulthood, becoming increasingly rare with decreasing age. The early onset of mood disorders is more apparent than in the past, but the most common time of onset is in adulthood. The anxiety disorders in this section and the adjustment disorders can begin at any age. Gender identity disorder is presumed to appear early in development, but may not become clinically apparent until much later. The sleep disorders are a heterogeneous group in time course and etiology.

■ EATING DISORDERS

Anorexia Nervosa

Clinical Description

Anorexia nervosa (AN) is characterized by a refusal to maintain normal weight or a failure to reach expected weight gain as a result of purposeful strict dieting or other extreme measures. Patients have either a distorted perception of their body shape and size or a denial of the seriousness of the weight loss. The preoccupation with food and body shape is obsessive. In severe cases, these patients may appear delusional. The appetite is not lost, rather there is an intense fear of gaining weight. Postmenarchal females cease menstruating. The *restricting type* of AN is characterized by strict dieting, fasting, or excessive exercise. In the *binge-eating/purging type,* huge quantities of food are eaten and then purged.

The physiological process of starvation leads to the development of additional psychological symptoms. Patients may become socially withdrawn, irritable, and anhedonic, with a decreased interest in sex, low self-esteem, and recurrent feelings of helplessness and inadequacy; this picture may be consistent with major depression. Depression impairs the individual's ability to function in the classroom, in social situations, and within the family. Patients tend to be controlling, not only of their own habits but also of those around them. Patients are often preoccupied with personal academic achievement and exercise. An accompanying diagnosis of obsessive-compulsive disorder (OCD) should be made if criteria are met.

Epidemiology

The majority of patients with AN are female, with an estimated prevalence of 0.5% of adolescent girls in the United States. Onset of AN prior to puberty is rare. The incidence peaks in the 15- to 24-year age group. Milder forms of eating disorders are even more common. AN is found predominantly in Western industrialized nations, and the prevalence is probably significantly affected by social and societal factors. The prevalence in boys, minority populations, and non-Western countries is lower but increasing.

Etiology

AN has a multifactorial etiology. Patients experience a variety of psychological, physical, academic, and social problems, although distinguishing cause and effect is often difficult. These patients tend to be dissatisfied with their bodies at puberty. Dieting is chosen as a socially acceptable method to improve the patient's sense of well-being and control.

Genetic and neurophysiological mechanisms contribute to the development of both AN and bulimia nervosa. First-degree relatives of anorexic and bulimic patients are 6–10 times more likely to have an eating disorder than are control populations. However, it remains difficult to separate environmental from heritable causative factors. Studies examining hormonal and neurohormonal relationships in adult and late adolescent eating disordered patients are promising. It is not clear whether these studies are identifying risk factors or simply measuring the effects of the disorder. For example, the hormone leptin has been implicated, but hormone levels often return to normal with refeeding and weight gain.

Although a history of sexual abuse may be present in patients with eating disorders, it is not clear that this risk is different from that in other psychiatric disorders, except perhaps for adolescents with bulimia. Family dynamics, including parental overinvolvement, lack of appropriate boundaries within the family, and insufficient autonomy, have received much attention in the literature, particularly from theorists such as Minuchin (Minuchin et al. 1978). However, few studies have tested these theories, and these characteristics are also present in families in which eating disorders do not develop. The effect on a family of having a child starving herself to death must not be confused with family characteristics that might have contributed to the disorder.

Course and Prognosis

AN usually presents during adolescence, between ages 14 and 18 years, a time of rapid growth with accompanying weight gain and changes in body shape. Although onset before puberty is less common, prepubertal children may develop AN or problem eating behaviors, including food avoidance, body image disturbance, inappropriate dieting, overeating, ritualistic behavior during meals, and selective eating. The first evidence of dissatisfaction with body shape may be found in a preoccupation with dieting. In one community survey, between one-half and two-thirds of all girls considered themselves to be overweight, although only 15% were actually overweight (Mellin et al. 1992).

Physiological changes are common. Medical complications may require hospitalization (Palla and Litt 1988; Table 5–1). The course of AN is typically prolonged, and the disorder does not remit without treatment. Continuing symptoms include low weight for height and age, peak bone mass reduction, excessive concern with weight or appearance, pubertal delay or interruption, amenorrhea, and troubled social and sexual relationships. Poor outcome is associated with longer duration of illness, extreme weight loss, and poor interpersonal relationships. Adolescent patients have a better prognosis, lower mortality, and better response to treatment than do adults.

Mortality in part depends on chronicity. Risk of death from medical complications of AN is estimated at between 5% and 6%, with some of these deaths due to suicide. Additional psychiatric diagnoses contribute to a poor prognosis, and partial remission rather than recovery and relapse are common, especially in those patients with psychiatric comorbidity.

Evaluation and Differential Diagnosis

A complete history, physical examination, and routine laboratory studies are necessary to rule out a medical cause for loss of weight or appetite. In addition, starvation can produce physiological disturbances that should be identified through laboratory studies (see Table 5–1). Hypoglycemia is a particularly poor prognostic sign. Dehydration can lead to elevations in blood urea nitrogen, liver function tests, and serum cholesterol levels. Signs of infection may be masked by leukopenia and hypothermia. Abnormal thyroid function studies are classified as "sick-euthyroid syndrome," with normal to low levels of thyroxine (T4) and free T4 and variable levels of thyroid-stimulating hormone.

The psychiatric interview of a patient with suspected AN includes details about the onset and course of the eating disorder, the highest and lowest weight, and the weight identified by the patient as most comfortable. The clinician should also explore daily eating patterns, including not only amounts of food but also times for meals. Questions about the use of laxatives, emetics, or diuretics can

TABLE 5–1. Physical signs and symptoms and complications associated with anorexia nervosa and bulimia nervosa

Cardiovascular	Hypotension (especially postural)
	Bradycardia (rates between 40 and 50 beats per minute)
	Arrhythmias (prolonged QT interval may be a marker for risk of sudden death)
	Mitral valve prolapse
	Cardiac arrest
	Edema and congestive heart failure during refeeding
	Cardiac failure secondary to cardiomyopathy from ipecac (emetine) poisoning
Neuroendocrine	Amenorrhea or irregular menses (low levels of FSH and LH despite low estrogen levels)
	Low basal metabolism rate
	Abnormal glucose tolerance test with insulin resistance
	Hypothermia
	Elevated levels of growth hormone and cortisol
	Sleep disturbances
Bone	Osteopenia
Fluid disturbance	Dehydration
	Electrolyte imbalance
	Abnormal urinalysis
Gastrointestinal	Constipation
	Diarrhea

TABLE 5–1. **Physical signs and symptoms and complications associated with anorexia nervosa and bulimia nervosa *(continued)***

Hematological	Leukopenia
	Anemia
	Thrombocytopenia
	Low sedimentation rate
Dermatological	Dry skin
	Lanugo (baby-fine body hair)
Oral, esophageal, and gastric damage from vomiting and/or binge eating	Loss of dental enamel
	Enlarged salivary glands
	Gastritis
	Esophagitis
	Esophageal tear
	Pancreatitis

Note.   FSH = follicle-stimulating hormone; LH = luteinizing hormone.
Source.   Adapted from Palla and Litt 1988.

be incorporated into this eating history. Although anorexic patients learn to disguise their continuing wish to lose weight, hide excessive exercise and purging, and claim to eat more than they do, they may inadvertently reveal important diagnostic information during an eating history.

In addition to individual assessments, a family evaluation is essential when treating young patients. The therapist may ask family members about their impressions of the illness and its origins. A review of at-home treatment attempts uncovers family dynamics and individual perceptions about the problem's origins and possible solutions. A family eating or weight history may show patterns of behavior imitated by the child or adolescent. Family history of psychiatric illness may suggest similar diagnoses in the patient.

The differential diagnosis of AN is shown in Table 5–2.

Treatment

The treatment of AN should be comprehensive and emphasize a return to normal eating patterns. In most cases, the initial focus of treatment is on acceptance of the disorder and weight gain. In severe cases, this initial phase may take place on an inpatient unit. Typical indications for inpatient hospitalization include weight more than 25%–30% below ideal body weight, rapid and severe weight loss refractory to outpatient treatment, symptomatic hypotension or syncope, heart rate below 50 beats per minute, or evidence of arrhythmia or a prolonged QTc interval. The denial of illness and fears of loss of control and of becoming fat generate severe resistance to treatment, even when the patient and family acknowledge the diagnosis. A firm focus on a target weight within 90% of the ideal body weight is helpful. The patient should reach this goal through gradual weight gain of 1 pound per week as an outpatient or 2–3 pounds per week while hospitalized (Mehler 2001). Too rapid increase in food intake can lead to medically dangerous "refeeding syndrome." Appetite stimulants are not recommended and may be contraindicated. Involvement of a primary care physician and a pediatric dietitian with experience in eating disorders is essential, whether treatment is inpatient or out-

TABLE 5–2. Differential diagnosis of anorexia nervosa

Normal thinness

Physical disorders causing weight loss

Hyperthyroidism

Other endocrine disorders

Gastrointestinal disorders resulting in vomiting, loss of appetite, and/or malabsorption

Malignancy

Chronic infection

Psychiatric disorders causing loss of appetite and weight loss

Depression

Peculiar eating behavior secondary to obsessive-compulsive disorder or to delusions in schizophrenia or psychotic depression

Avoidance of eating caused by phobia of choking, with or without psychosis

Vomiting secondary to conversion disorder

Hypothyroidism producing hypothermia and amenorrhea

patient. Psychotherapeutic approaches can act as an adjunct to the re-feeding regimen. Forced weight gain alone is futile, and too-rapid weight gain exacerbates fears of loss of control and may be medically hazardous. Tube or intravenous feeding is reserved for medical emergencies, because these methods are viewed by patients as punitive. The patient's sabotage of these methods can be dangerous (e.g., bleeding from the site of a pulled intravenous line, aspiration of tube feedings). Regardless of the success of refeeding, a comprehensive treatment plan that includes an exploration of underlying psychological factors is essential.

Family therapy is particularly effective when symptoms appeared prior to age 18. The Maudsley model of family-based treatment has empirical support (Lock et al. 2005). Families are affected secondarily by the presence of the eating disorder, and the clinician should not assume that every family has premorbid problems. Psycho-educational programs for family members greatly facilitate treatment and may be done in an individual or group setting. Family involvement in treatment, whatever the primary modality, clearly benefits young patients. Current family-based treatment emphasizes parents as part of the solution, not the cause of the problem.

Behavior modification facilitates an initial gain to a minimal healthy weight, which decreases the medical risk and the negative emotional and behavioral effects of starvation. Privileges and activities are made contingent on weight gain. The benefits of this intervention appear to be short lived, however. Cognitive-behavioral modification initially emphasizes changing incorrect beliefs and dysfunctional cognitions about food and eating. The focus of treatment eventually extends to include issues of body weight, appearance, peer relationships, and individual control. Cognitive-behavioral interventions (e.g., the use of food diaries) have been effective, particularly in preventing relapse in patients whose weight had returned to normal.

Individual psychotherapy is generally a second choice for adolescent patients but may be indicated for patients whose families are unwilling or unable to participate. Once the patient's eating patterns have normalized, interpersonal psychotherapies may provide insight for the patient that will facilitate long-term recovery. Older patients tend to do well with individual therapies, while younger patients respond best to family interventions.

There is little evidence regarding the use of medication in the treatment of AN. Adjunctive atypical antipsychotic medication (such as olanzapine) may decrease anxiety, improve sleep, decrease obsessional rumination, and aid in weight gain. However, these medications can contribute to the initiation of bingeing behavior, and no controlled studies exist on their efficacy or safety. Although not systematically studied, selective serotonin reuptake inhibitors (SSRIs) may assist with comorbid anxiety and depression, once weight has stabilized.

Bulimia Nervosa

Clinical Description

Bulimia nervosa (BN) is characterized by repeated episodes of uncontrollable binge eating of huge amounts of food in a short time (2-hour period) accompanied by excessive attempts to compensate for this caloric intake. Bingeing and compensatory behaviors occur at least twice a week for at least 3 months. Binge eating is typically done secretly and may initially be pleasurable. The patient may engage in the behavior during a dysphoric episode or in response to a recent stressor. The binge usually brings the patient relief, but self-deprecatory thoughts return. Patients feel that their eating is out of control.

Exercise and strict fasting are the most common compensatory behaviors, followed by induced vomiting. The use of laxatives, enemas, diuretics, or thyroid medication is less common, particularly in the pediatric population.

Adolescent patients increase the frequency of binges as the disorder develops. Patients with BN are generally of normal weight but may be slightly over or under their ideal weight, and may be prone to obesity before the onset of the disorder. The patient's self-image is unduly influenced by body shape and weight.

Epidemiology

Studies on the prevalence of BN are affected by changing diagnostic criteria, the short history of the diagnosis, and the secrecy of the behavior. BN is more common than AN. Almost 50% of cases appear before age 18 years. Binge eating is common among adolescents, but relatively few meet diagnostic criteria for BN. Approximately 1%–2% of adolescent females and 0.2% of adolescent males in the United States have BN. Males account for 10%–15% of all clinically referred patients with BN. Patients generally become ill in the latter half of adolescence. Risk is increased in elite athletes whose sport emphasizes thinness or ballet dancers. Bulimic patients have increased rates of drug and alcohol use, tend to be of higher socioeconomic status, and are typically white or Hispanic. Recent studies have noted an increasing prevalence of BN and purging with laxatives in the African American population, although the prevalence is still lower than in whites or Latinas. Dysfunctional behaviors related to eating and weight are relatively common among adolescent and young adult females, with many meeting criteria for a diagnosis of eating disorder not otherwise specified. Studies of adolescent females note that between 40% and 60% are "dieting" to lose weight. This is particularly true among white adolescent girls from high-income families. In more than 10% of these, dieting may include induced vomiting or the use of diet pills and diuretics. Dieting behavior clearly increases the risk for eating disorders.

Etiology

AN and BN frequently present on a continuum, and many patients demonstrate symptoms of each. Approximately 50% of patients with AN will develop bulimic symptoms, and up to a quarter of patients with BN become anorectic. Identical twins of patients with BN have higher rates of the disorder. Monozygotic twins have higher concordance rates than do dizygotic twins. A family history of obesity, depression, or alcoholism is common. Serotonin has become a focus in studies of BN. Sexual and physical abuse predispose children to various psychiatric disorders but not preferentially to the development of eating disorders.

Course and Prognosis

Dieting usually precedes the development of BN. The patient first begins to binge-eat as a direct result of food restriction; the behavior then becomes a compulsion or an addiction. The patient regards bingeing as abhorrent behavior, which contributes to feelings of depression and self-criticism. The patient once again begins dieting, often augmented with vigorous exercise or purging, in an attempt to undo the damage of the binge. Although these behaviors give the patient temporary relief from the emotional pain, they become part of a vicious cycle that maintains symptoms of BN and depression. A constant state of semistarvation results, which places the patient at additional risk for mood disorders.

Few studies have examined either the short- or the long-term prognosis for treated bulimic patients. Relapse rates are 30%–50% when patients are followed for 6 months to 6 years. Some speculate that improvement continues for 10–15 years. Risk factors for relapse include induced vomiting and the use of alcohol or drugs. Patients with milder symptoms at the onset of treatment appear to have a better prognosis. Among bulimic adolescents, comorbid anxiety or mood disorders predict continued eating-disordered behaviors. No factors have been identified as predictive of treatment success. Studies note a BN mortality rate of approximately 5%.

Social complications can be severe, with time and finances depleted by obtaining food, binge eating, and purging. School functioning and peer relationships typically deteriorate. Associated disorders include depression, substance abuse, and (in adults) borderline personality disorder. The presence of a comorbid medical diagnosis (i.e., diabetes, cystic fibrosis) may cause otherwise benign levels of symptoms to become dangerous. The risk of suicide or death from medical complications is significant. Risk factors for death from bulimia include a greater than 2-year duration; daily vomiting or bingeing; and use of laxatives, diuretics, ipecac, and stimulants (diet pills).

Evaluation and Differential Diagnosis

The clinician should evaluate the patient by 1) obtaining a detailed lifetime history of weight changes, noting periods of greatest fluctuation; 2) inquiring about current eating patterns in a typical day, including the number of calories consumed and any use of diet pills; 3) determining the onset and current status of bingeing and purging behaviors; and 4) asking about possible use of thyroid hormone, excessive exercise, laxatives, and diuretics. The medical history may suggest a neurological, endocrinological, or genetic (e.g., Prader-Willi syndrome) etiology of binge eating. Patients may have medical complications (see Table 5–1). The abuse of laxatives can lead to abdominal cramping, diarrhea, or rectal bleeding. Vomiting or abuse of diuretics or laxatives can produce metabolic alkalosis, elevations in serum amylase, hypomagnesemia and hypophosphatemia, and hypokalemia. A review of psychiatric history focuses on comorbidity and on previous treatment attempts. The individual's social and personal history may reveal contributing factors. Family assessment considers dynamics; previous attempts to help the patient; eating habits; and a review of significant social, medical, and psychiatric family history.

Treatment

Goals of treatment include eliminating the binge–purge cycle, establishing healthy eating habits, and promoting new strategies and skills to deal with emotions and problematic situations. The treatment plan progresses in a stepwise fashion, beginning with nutritional rehabilitation. Nutritional consultation can facilitate eating regular, well-balanced meals to avoid the hunger that triggers the urge to binge. Patients with BN who maintain a normal weight generally do not require hospitalization. Hospitalization is indicated when the patient is suicidal, has out-of-control eating and vomiting, is metabolically unstable, or does not respond to outpatient treatment. In the hospital, a behavior contract can be implemented, with activities and privileges contingent on eating regular meals and not vomiting.

Patients must be watched closely for hiding or stealing food and for secretive vomiting.

Cognitive-behavioral modification is the most effective treatment for BN in adults. Case series and one controlled trial support its use in adolescents (Schmidt et al. 2007). It can help patients overcome feelings of helplessness and the habit of using food to deal with their uncomfortable feelings. The patient learns skills and strategies for problem solving, coping with stress, identifying feelings, and avoiding relapse. Patients are more successful when they have lower weights and do not abuse laxatives or diuretics. Family therapy appears to be particularly effective in the adolescent population. A manualized family-based treatment for BN in adolescents has empirical support (Le Grange et al. 2007).

Pharmacological treatment of BN in adults uses SSRIs, but evidence of benefit when an SSRI is added to CBT is lacking. Pharmacological treatment of BN in adolescents is not as effective as cognitive-behavioral approaches. Bupropion is associated with the occurrence of grand mal seizures and should not be used in these patients. The SSRIs (e.g., fluoxetine) may be effective.

■ SUBSTANCE-RELATED DISORDERS

Clinical Description

The DSM-IV-TR criteria for the substance-related disorders do not change with age. The continuum of adolescent substance use ranges from nonusers, through experimental and casual users, to abuse and dependence. The line between use and abuse is crossed more easily by young persons than by adults, and some recommend that any use of alcohol or illicit drugs among people under the legal drinking age be called abuse. Although any use of substances by an adolescent constitutes risk-taking behavior, DSM-IV-TR requires evidence of harmful consequences for a diagnosis of abuse. Physical dependence is rare in adolescents.

Epidemiology

Two national surveys provide regularly updated data on substance use in youth. The National Institute on Drug Abuse (NIDA)–sponsored Monitoring the Future survey is an ongoing study of the behaviors, attitudes, and values of American secondary school students, college students, and young adults. Each year, approximately 50,000 8th-, 10th-, and 12th-grade students are surveyed (report available at http://monitoringthefuture.org). The reported rates are likely underestimates, because many of the heaviest drug users drop out of school or are likely to be absent when surveys are taken. The National Survey on Drug Use and Health (NSDUH), conducted by the Substance Abuse and Mental Health Services Administration (SAMHSA), uses an interactive, computer-based questionnaire to provide annual reports on the prevalence, patterns, and consequences of drug and alcohol use and abuse in the general U.S. civilian noninstitutionalized population ages 12 years and older (report available at http://www.drugabusestatistics.samhsa.gov).

The 2009 NSDUH data show overall illicit drug use in 12- to 17-year-olds at 10%, slightly higher than in 2008. Tobacco use and drinking remained stable, but the rate of marijuana use increased, with use in 2009 at 7.3%. Even more concerning is the drop in the number of teens who perceive great harm in frequent marijuana use—less than half of those surveyed.

The 2010 Monitoring the Future survey found that the substantial decrease in teen smoking since the mid-1990s has plateaued and the rate of smoking may be increasing. Eleven percent of 12th graders reported daily smoking in the past month. In addition, negative attitudes about smoking and smokers, at a peak in 2007, have leveled off or begun to decline. Over the past several years the use of smokeless tobacco has increased, following a decline from the mid-1990s to the early 2000s. New concerns on the horizon are hookah water pipes and small cigars.

In the 2010 Monitoring the Future data, 16% of surveyed eighth graders reported using an illicit drug in the past year, up from 14.5% in 2009. Compared with the previous year, fewer teens report believing that marijuana or Ecstasy is risky to use. Marijuana is the most commonly used illicit drug among youth. Use of Ecstasy is low but increasing again, and abuse of prescription drugs continues. There is some abuse of stimulants and sedatives, but most worrying is non-medical use of opiates like OxyContin and Vicodin. Use of cocaine continues to decline, and prevalence is far lower than in the mid-1980s. Inhalant and LSD use continues, and the proportion of teens who consider their use to be dangerous has declined since 2001. As many as 6.6% of surveyed 12th graders report past-year use of cough and cold medicine to get high. Use of alcohol and prevalence of binge drinking continue to decline from the peak in the late 1990s.

A new concern is *Salvia divinorum,* a plant whose leaves can be smoked, chewed, or brewed, for a brief hallucinatory or dissociative experience. Many states have banned or restricted its sale, but it remains relatively easily available.

Comorbidity

Virtually all adolescents referred for treatment of substance use have additional disorders, including attention-deficit/hyperactivity disorder (ADHD), oppositional defiant disorder (ODD), conduct disorder (CD), depression, anxiety disorders, posttraumatic stress disorder (PTSD), psychosis, and specific developmental disorders (learning disabilities). Virtually any psychiatric disorder may occur in association with substance use as a cause, an effect, or a correlate. Psychiatric disorders may predate substance abuse or be secondary to pharmacological or situational effects of drug use. In a longitudinal school-based study of adolescents, major depression and heavy smoking each increased the prospective risk for the other. This association does not appear to be due to shared risk factors (Windle and Windle 2001). The presence of ADHD, especially when accompanied by ODD or CD, is associated with early onset of substance abuse.

Etiology

Children of substance abusers appear to be particularly vulnerable to adolescent drug use, likely resulting from a combination of ge-

TABLE 5–3.	Risk factors associated with serious substance abuse in adolescence

Rebelliousness
Aggression
Impulsivity
Low self-esteem
Elementary school underachievement
Failure to value education
Absence of strong religious convictions
Experimentation with drugs before age 15 years
Relationships with peers who have behavior problems and
  use drugs
Alienation from parents
History of physical or sexual abuse
Family lacking in clear discipline, praise, and positive relationships
Family history of substance abuse

netic and family dynamic factors with learned attitudes toward substance use (Table 5–3). Genetic contributions to alcoholism are strongest in males. Peer influence mediates avoidance of drugs, as well as both initiation and maintenance of substance use. Substances may be used to produce positive feelings and avoid unpleasant ones, relieve tension and stress, reduce disturbing emotions, alleviate depression or anxiety, and gain peer acceptance. Among youth, determinants of use are often specific to each drug, related to some extent to the perceived risks and benefits of the substance.

Course and Prognosis

Adolescence is the critical period for initiation of drug abuse. Onset is rare in adulthood, except for the abuse of prescription drugs. Substance abuse typically progresses in predictable stages (Kandel 1975). Each stage serves as a "gateway" to the next—from abstinence to cigarettes, then beer or wine, to hard liquor, to marijuana, and then to other illicit drugs. At each stage, many youths do not progress further, but when progression occurs, stages are rarely skipped. Almost all adolescents who have tried cocaine and heroin first used alcohol, tobacco, and cannabis. The earlier cannabis use is begun and the more often cannabis is used, the more likely is progression to other illicit drugs. In general, drugs from each stage are continued into the next, leading to a pattern of multiple drug abuse. Abuse of inhalants is an exception. Children may begin to use these easily available volatile substances (e.g., glue, freon, propane, aerosols, paint thinner, lighter fluid, gasoline, nitrous oxide, butane, amyl and butyl nitrite) but then desist as they gain access to other drugs. Although many young people experiment with alcohol and drugs, a smaller number proceed to regular use, and only a fraction of those become chemically dependent. Unfortunately, it is difficult to predict which young people will only experiment with substances or continue social use of alcohol, in contrast to those who will progress to chemical dependency. Early onset and rapid progression appear to increase the risk for subsequent serious problems.

In children and adolescents, substance use interferes with developing cognitive, social, and physical abilities. Chronic use of marijuana may result in apathy and resulting arrest of academic and social development. Critical developmental experiences that are missed may be difficult or impossible to replace, leading to high risk for impairment of future functioning in every sphere. Potential morbidity and mortality from substance use are substantial. Rates of suicidal ideation and behavior are increased. The risk of death from intentional or accidental overdose, dangerous behavior while intoxicated (especially automobile accidents), or homicide related to drug dealing is significant. Injection drug use is the current major vehicle for the spread of human immunodeficiency virus (HIV) among adolescents. Hepatitis is also a risk. Indiscriminate sexual activity (related to direct drug effect on impulse control and judgment or induced by prostitution to buy drugs) places the adolescent at high risk for exposure to HIV and other sexually transmitted diseases. Adolescent female drug users may become pregnant and place the developing fetus at risk for drug-induced damage or HIV infection. Inhalant abuse may result in brain damage, cardiac arrest, liver and kidney damage, or lead poisoning.

Evaluation and Differential Diagnosis

A high index of suspicion for substance use is essential in all clinical settings. Virtually any change in emotional state, behavior, social activities, or academic performance can signal a problem with substance use. The clinician should question all patients older than 9 years about substance use in a nonjudgmental manner. If there is evidence of substance use, the patient should be asked about every category of substance, including details of amount, frequency, impairment, and social and emotional context. Verification by parents, teachers, other professionals, or peers may be crucial. Specific areas of inquiry should include intoxication at school, missing classes because of substance use, evidence of tolerance, and preferences among drugs that indicate experience. Sequelae of substance use, such as decline in school attendance or grades, increase in family conflict, cessation of previously important activities, association with a marginal peer group, and involvement in risky behavior (especially driving while intoxicated and reckless sexual behavior), should be specifically queried, as well as motivation and any attempts to decrease or stop use.

Self-report questionnaires are available for use with adolescents, including the Drug Use Screening Inventory (DUSI) (Tarter 1990), the Drug and Alcohol Problem (DAP) Quick Screen (Schwartz and Wirtz 1990), and the CAGE (Dias 2002).

Because most young substance users have "dual diagnoses" (psychiatric disorders in addition to substance use disorders), it is helpful to attempt to establish the chronology of substance use with respect to the emotional and behavioral symptoms. A detailed family history of psychiatric disorders and substance use is essential. The risk of substance abuse in parents and siblings is high.

Physical or neurological examination may disclose effects of substance use. Physical signs and symptoms of inhalant abuse may include spots or sores around the mouth, red or runny eyes or nose, dazed or dizzy appearance, and nausea or loss of appetite. Laboratory screening for drug use can provide valuable information, although false-positive and false-negative results occur, and verification and integration with the rest of the assessment are essential.

Treatment

The primary goal is achieving and maintaining abstinence. Medical detoxification is rarely necessary in adolescents. Common features of treatment programs for substance abuse include developmentally appropriate approaches to abstinence, group therapy with other substance abusers, participation in self-help "12-Step" programs such as Alcoholics Anonymous (AA) and Narcotics Anonymous (NA), and the concept of "recovery" rather than cure. The effects of denial, lack of motivation, and the peer drug culture make conventional individual psychotherapy unlikely to succeed. Better response to treatment may be associated with motivation and cooperation in the patient and family, the patient's willingness to undergo urine testing, earlier stages of drug use, and remaining in treatment longer. Suggested therapeutic interventions include using motivational interviewing techniques; teaching social skills and strategies for problem solving, coping, and relapse prevention; and encouraging structured and supervised recreational activities with drug-free peers. Comorbid psychiatric disorders and specific learning disorders must be addressed and treated, although they cannot be validly assessed without a period of abstinence. Academic deficits need to be remedied, and vocational testing and training may be useful for older adolescents for whom return to school is unlikely.

Family therapy approaches have been shown to be effective, particularly those that use structural and behavioral techniques to address parent–youth relationships and interaction patterns, as well as behavior management skills training for parents. Other effective models add interventions with peers, teachers, and other parts of the youth's social environment, as well as job and school skills training for youth (Henggeler et al. 2002).

Short-term hospitalization (5–30 days) is now used primarily when outpatient treatment has failed or comorbidity with other psychiatric conditions increases the acute risk of harm to self or others. Both the patient and the family should be actively involved in group treatment and education regarding drugs. Psychotropic medications may alleviate concomitant disorders, reduce withdrawal symptoms, or facilitate abstinence. Residential treatment for 3 to 12 months is used only for the most severe, complex, or recalcitrant cases or when a parent is an active drug user.

Long-term continuation of treatment is important as an outpatient or in a day treatment program or halfway house. Intensive participation in AA or NA is often required. Adolescents generally do best in groups with other adolescents rather than mixed with adults. Family therapy is an integral part of treatment. Goals include educating parents about substance abuse and its consequences, thus decreasing denial and facilitating their support of treatment and of abstinence; improving parental skills of firm and consistent, but supportive, limit setting and supervision; and enhancing communication between family members. Parents may require referral for treatment of their own substance use or other psychiatric disorders. Effective treatment results in less substance abuse as well as improved school performance and fewer behavioral and psychological symptoms.

Relapses are common and should be viewed as predictable complications rather than as catastrophes or reasons for terminating treatment. Relapse prevention (i.e., specific attention to situations in which drug use is likely, with training in coping strategies) may reduce the number and severity of relapses. Periodic urine testing can facilitate abstinence.

■ SCHIZOPHRENIA

Clinical Description

DSM-IV-TR criteria for schizophrenia do not change with age, except that in children, failure to reach expected levels of interpersonal or academic functioning may be seen instead of deterioration. Schizophrenia in children is characterized by markedly uneven development and gradual onset. Language and social behavior not only are delayed but also are qualitatively different from those seen in nonschizophrenic children at any developmental stage. Peers rapidly identify schizophrenic children as different. Visual hallucinations are more common in children with schizophrenia than in adults. Delusions and hallucinations may be less complex than those in adults.

120

Epidemiology

Childhood-onset schizophrenia (COS) (i.e., onset before age 13 years) is quite rare. Prevalence prior to adolescence is less than 0.1%. It is somewhat more common in boys than in girls. After puberty, the prevalence increases and approaches adult levels (1%) in late adolescence.

Etiology

Schizophrenia is considered to be a neurodevelopmental disorder. A substantial genetic contribution is evident, and various prenatal neurological insults have been implicated. There is no evidence that psychological or social factors cause schizophrenia.

Course and Prognosis

COS typically has an insidious onset and chronic course. Common premorbid symptoms are language and motor delays; academic problems; short attention span, hyperactivity, and disruptive behavior; social withdrawal and isolation; and symptoms usually associated with pervasive developmental disorder, such as echolalia, rituals, and stereotypies. The course appears to be similar to that in chronic poor-outcome adult schizophrenia. In schizophrenia with adolescent onset, premorbid social, motor, and language impairments are often present. Some adolescents have episodes and remissions like those seen in some adults. The range of outcomes for adolescent-onset schizophrenia appears to be similar to that for adult-onset schizophrenia, and most patients remain impaired in social relationships and educational or job skills that would permit independent living. Adolescents with schizophrenia are at increased risk for death from suicide or accidents.

Evaluation and Differential Diagnosis

A careful history is necessary to clarify premorbid functioning and current positive (e.g., delusions, hallucinations) and negative (e.g., apathy, affective flattening, poverty of speech) symptoms. A history of sexual or physical abuse may identify the precipitant of acute symptoms or suggest an alternative diagnosis (e.g., PTSD). In adolescents, a detailed drug and alcohol use history and a urine drug test are needed. The clinician should ascertain the presence and nature of command hallucinations and suicidal ideation. Comorbid disorders should be identified.

Pediatric and neurological evaluations are required to rule out organic psychoses, both acute (delirium or intoxication) and chronic. Causes include brain tumor; congenital malformation; head trauma; seizure disorder; neurodegenerative disorder; metabolic disorder; toxic encephalopathy due to substance abuse, prescribed medication (e.g., stimulants, corticosteroids, anticholinergic agents), or other toxins such as heavy metals; and infections (encephalitis or HIV-related syndromes). The extent of the medical and neurological workup and any neuroimaging or electroencephalography should be guided by the clinical history and neurological examination.

When a psychotic child or adolescent first presents clinically, the clinician often has difficulty making a definitive diagnosis. One of the most difficult distinctions is between schizophrenia and *bipolar disorder with psychosis*. Longitudinal follow-up and periodic reassessment are essential, and a family history may be helpful. Thought disorder is difficult to diagnose prior to age 7 years. In young children who are nonverbal, it is not possible to diagnose schizophrenia. Some of these children appear to have *autistic disorder* or other *pervasive developmental disorder*. As the child develops language, evidence of delusions, hallucinations, and thought disorder emerges, enabling the correct diagnosis to be made. True autistic disorder does not "change into" classic schizophrenia, although very rarely both may be present. Among children referred for presumed COS, a substantial proportion do not actually meet DSM criteria, but instead have been characterized as *multidimensionally impaired* (McKenna et al. 1994). Their condition does not fit into any of the existing diagnostic categories, but they have a variety of impairing psychiatric symptoms, including poor reality testing, perceptual disturbances, neuropsychological deficits, affective instability, and inability to relate to peers despite attempts to do so.

Most children who have hallucinations are not schizophrenic. Acute hallucinations occur in nonschizophrenic children as a result of *acute phobic reactions, physical illness with fever or metabolic aberration, migraine headaches,* or *medications.* Recurring hallucinations may appear in *dissociative disorder, PTSD, mania,* and *major depressive disorder.* In young children, it may be difficult to differentiate delusions and hallucinations from fantasy play or magical thinking at the extreme end of the normal range, or from play with normal imaginary companions. Children may have difficulty distinguishing between psychotic hallucinations and dreams, illusions, and hallucinations occurring while falling asleep (hypnagogic) or awakening (hypnopompic). Apparent delusions or hallucinations may also be reflections of shared religious or cultural beliefs.

Mental retardation is manifested by multiple delays in development without the peculiarities of thought and behavior characteristic of schizophrenia. The two disorders may be comorbid, however. Apparent thought disorder may actually be *deafness* or *language disorder.* Adolescents with *schizotypal* or *borderline personality disorder* have severe symptoms that may resemble schizophrenia, but they do not have hallucinations or delusions. Inattention and distractibility may be present, but DSM-IV-TR specifies that *ADHD* is not diagnosed in the presence of schizophrenia. Other differential diagnostic possibilities include *schizophreniform disorder, brief psychotic disorder, schizoaffective disorder, organic syndromes, intoxication or withdrawal due to substance abuse, OCD,* and *depression with psychotic features.*

Treatment

The treatment plan should be comprehensive and reevaluated at regular intervals. The cornerstone of treatment is an intensive program that includes a structured environment, programming in school or day treatment tailored to the child's needs, and social skills training. Treatment must address developmental arrests and regression, as well as specific symptoms of schizophrenia and any comorbid conditions. Hospitalization or long-term residential treatment may be needed, but less so than in the past. Community support services include crisis intervention, respite care, and in-home interventions for the child and family. Family, individual, or group psychoeducational treatment is important and can reduce the rate and severity of relapse. Advocacy groups such as the National Alliance for the Mentally Ill Child and Adolescent Network (NAMI-CAN) can provide support to families and concrete assistance with accessing resources.

Supportive individual psychotherapy may be useful as a part of a comprehensive treatment plan. The therapist must be prepared to provide structure, to limit regression and fantasy, and to focus on reality testing and development of stronger defense mechanisms and healthier coping skills. The relationship with the therapist may be especially crucial for these youngsters.

Medication (see Chapter 8) is indicated as part of the treatment program if positive psychotic symptoms cause significant impairment or interfere with other interventions. Target symptoms that may respond include overactivity, aggression, agitation, stereotyped movements, delusions, and hallucinations. Full efficacy may not appear for many months. Disabling negative symptoms (e.g., apathy and social withdrawal) also may be indications for treatment with an atypical antipsychotic, but degree of improvement is often disappointing. In general, adolescents with schizophrenia are less responsive to pharmacotherapy than are adults and continue to have substantial impairment, even if the more florid symptoms abate. Prepubertal children are less likely to respond to antipsychotics, and these children are more likely to have troublesome sedation. The risk of tardive dyskinesia or metabolic syndrome mandates caution in the prescription of antipsychotic drugs. Based on the limited pediatric research to date, risperidone, quetiapine, or aripiprazole is often the initial medication choice.

■ MOOD DISORDERS

Clinical Description

DSM-IV-TR criteria for mood disorders are the same for children and adults, with a few exceptions (Table 5–4). At all ages, depressed

TABLE 5–4.   Developmental differences in DSM-IV-TR
              criteria for mood disorders

Disorder	Adults	Children
Major depression	Depressed mood	Can be irritable mood
	Change in weight or appetite	Can be failure to make expected weight gains
Dysthymia	Depressed mood	Can be irritable mood
	2-year duration	1-year duration
Cyclothymia	2-year duration	1-year duration

mood inferred from observation of the patient (appears sad or tear-
ful) can be substituted for the patient's report. The anhedonia criterion of diminished interest or pleasure in activities can be met by
observed apathy. Children and adolescents often report this as pervasive boredom. Mood-related symptoms may be manifested in different ways at different developmental levels. Key indicators of
depression in young people are declining school performance, withdrawal from social activities, somatic symptoms (especially headaches and abdominal pain), sleep difficulties, and conduct problems.
Consistent neurovegetative symptoms are rare in childhood depression or dysthymic disorder. Of the criteria for the diagnosis of mania, children have far less opportunity than adults for buying sprees
or foolish investments. The classic pattern of alternating episodes of
depressed and elated mood with corresponding vegetative (sleep,
activity, appetite) symptoms does not typically emerge until late
adolescence or adulthood.

Epidemiology

The prevalence of major depression has been estimated at 1%–3% in
prepubertal children and 3%–9% in adolescents, although rates vary
with the population, the diagnostic criteria, and the methods of assessment. In the Oregon Adolescent Depression Project, Lewinsohn
and colleagues (1994) found the lifetime prevalence of at least one
episode of major depression by late adolescence to be 20%–25% and

of dysthymic disorder to be 3%. Many more youth have depressive symptoms than have full major depression or dysthymia. Before puberty, depression is equally common in boys and girls, with a change in adolescence to the female predominance found in adults.

Mania is rare before middle adolescence but by late adolescence is nearly as common as in adults. A community survey of high school students found a lifetime prevalence of 1% for all bipolar disorders. An additional 5.7% of the sample had persistent subthreshold hypomanic and associated symptoms (Lewinsohn et al. 1995). Approximately 20% of all bipolar patients have their first episode during adolescence.

Etiology

Etiological factors for mood disorders in children are similar to those in adults. Depression in a parent may be a powerful contributing factor to depression in young people, via genetic transmission, plus the parent's modeling, emotional unavailability, and decreased capacity for parenting. Abuse and neglect may be significant precipitants, especially in very young children.

Course and Prognosis

Mood disorders in childhood are serious and potentially fatal problems. In a 15-year follow-up of children with major depression, 4% had died by suicide (Wolk and Weissman 1996). A 10- to 15-year follow-up of a clinical sample of subjects with adolescent onset of major depression found that nearly 8% had committed suicide (Weissman et al. 1999). Over the full age range, earlier age at onset implies a lengthier and more severe course and greater genetic loading. Over the past 25 years, the age at onset of major depression appears to have decreased. In a prospective study of clinically referred prepubertal children, the median length of the major depressive episode was 9 months. The median length of time for recovery from dysthymia was 4 years. Dysthymia often progressed to a major depressive episode before resolving. Risk for subsequent episodes of major depression or dysthymia is high (Kovacs 1996). In a sample of high school students, episodes of major depression lasted as long as 10 years (mean=26 weeks; median=8 weeks). Of those who recovered, one-third had another episode within 4 years. Suicidal ideation was associated with earlier onset, longer episodes, and earlier relapse of depression (Lewinsohn et al. 1994). Follow-up studies of depressed youth consistently find increased risk of repeated mood disorders and other psychiatric disorders and impairment in subsequent educational and vocational achievement and peer and family relationships.

Childhood-onset depression is more likely than adult-onset depression to evolve into bipolar disorder. Among adolescents with major depression, subsequent bipolar mood disorder was predicted by precipitous onset of symptoms, psychomotor retardation, psychotic features, psychopharmacologically precipitated hypomania, and family history of bipolar disorder (Strober and Carlson 1982).

Evaluation and Differential Diagnosis

The clinician should ask children direct questions about depression. Young children have more difficulty recognizing and verbalizing their feelings and may use idiosyncratic words to describe dysphoria or anhedonia. Both parent and child reports are essential. Some children report their mood states more accurately than their parents can, although young children may have limited insight into other symptoms. A trained clinician should observe children for depressed affect. The Children's Depression Inventory (CDI) (Kovacs 1985) may be a useful self-report screening instrument.

Assessment of the degree of potentially dangerous behavior is crucial. The clinician can question children directly regarding suicidal ideation, plans, and attempts. No evidence indicates that inquiries about wishes to die increase the risk of self-destructive behavior. Substance abuse increases the risk of suicide. (See Chapter 7 for discussion of suicidal behavior.) The clinician should ask specifically about emotional or physical abuse or neglect of the child.

The characteristics and prevalence of pediatric bipolar (manic-depressive) disorder are controversial, especially prior to puberty. Youth seem more often to have mixed episodes without clear cycling accompanied by changes in sleep, appetite, and energy, and are more prone to rapid cycling than are adults. Patients who meet adult criteria for bipolar disorder may be considered to have the *narrow phenotype,* while those characterized more by chronic severe explosive irritability and aggression (*broad phenotype*) may be considered to have *severe mood dysregulation.* The correlates and course of severe mood dysregulation appear to be different from those of classic bipolar disorder.

Mania and hypomania occurring before adulthood are often misdiagnosed or not recognized. Children and adolescents with bipolar disorder are prone to a chronic mixed state or rapid cycling, with dysphoric, agitated affect and explosive anger. Heedless risk taking, highly energized affect, and developmentally inappropriate sexual preoccupation and behavior are useful markers for mania. Precocious sexuality in a child with manic symptoms should not be presumed to be evidence of sexual abuse. Grandiosity is expressed in different terms than in adults, but the experienced clinician can distinguish these beliefs from normal bragging or childhood fantasy (Geller et al. 2002a). Manic or hypomanic decreased need for sleep must be differentiated from insomnia, resistance to bedtime, or substance use. Family history and longitudinal course may provide important clues.

Anxiety disorders, ADHD, or disruptive behavior disorders frequently coexist with depression, dysthymia, or bipolar disorder, even in nonclinical community epidemiological samples. Their onset may precede or follow the onset of the mood disorder. Alcohol or drug abuse may cause a secondary depression or may represent an attempt to "self-medicate" dysphoria. Diagnosis of a mood disorder may be impossible without observing the patient in a drug-free state. *Separation anxiety disorder* may resemble major depression or dysthymic disorder or may coexist with it. Children younger than 4 years may develop a clinical picture similar to major depression when separated from their parents. Children with *reac-*

tive attachment disorder secondary to parental abuse or neglect who present with lethargy, apathy, and withdrawal may appear depressed.

Both mania and agitated depression may be confused with *ADHD,* but mood disorders are typically episodic, whereas ADHD is a chronic condition with onset in early childhood. Symptoms that best discriminate juvenile bipolar disorder from ADHD are elation, grandiosity, flight of ideas/racing thoughts, decreased need for sleep, and hypersexuality (Geller et al. 2002b). Mania in childhood and adolescence is frequently misdiagnosed as *schizophrenia.* Manic or depressed youth may have some symptoms of *ODD* or *CD* that are secondary to their mood symptoms. Of course, *disruptive behavior disorder* may precede mood disorder or develop in parallel. *Secondary mania* may result from prescribed medication (e.g., steroids, carbamazepine, antidepressants, stimulants), illegal drugs (e.g., cocaine, amphetamines), metabolic abnormalities (especially hyperthyroidism), or central nervous system disturbances (e.g., tumor, trauma, multiple sclerosis, epilepsy, infections).

The strong family clustering of mood disorders suggests that parents and siblings should be evaluated routinely for mood and anxiety disorders, and treatment should be provided or arranged as necessary.

Treatment

If risk-taking behavior or suicidal ideation is present, close parental and psychiatric supervision is needed. Psychiatric hospitalization may be required for youngsters who are psychotic or seriously suicidal or who do not respond to outpatient treatment.

Early-onset mood disorders often have devastating effects on development. Long-term treatment is often needed. Even after spontaneous remission or successful treatment, reduced coping skills, cognitive patterns associated with depression, and impaired interpersonal relationships with peers and family members may require individual, group, or family therapy to address developmental deficits or sequelae of the depression. Whatever the treatment, involvement of the family is even more crucial than for adult patients. Both patients and families benefit from psychoeducational therapy (provision of information about the disorder and its treatment) (see Appendix) and from instruction in relapse prevention (complying with medication, recognizing early symptoms of relapse, and avoiding precipitants of relapse such as sleep deprivation and drug abuse). Up to 60% of patients with mild to moderate depression respond to supportive treatment.

Fluoxetine (age 8 years and older) and escitalopram (age 12 years and older) are currently approved by the U.S. Food and Drug Administration (FDA) for the treatment of pediatric major depressive disorder. For nonpsychotic depression, psychotherapy is typically the first treatment. Medication is added if symptoms do not improve in 4–6 weeks. For more severe depression, medication is indicated as initial treatment. Cognitive-behavioral therapy (CBT) and interpersonal therapy (IPT) techniques developed for the treatment of depression in adults have been adapted for use in children and adolescents (Mufson et al. 2004) (see also "Additional Reading"). Social withdrawal and limited peer relationships may respond to behavior modification and social skills training. Remedial education or tutoring may be needed when the illness has interfered with learning in school.

A clinical-consensus empirically informed algorithm suggests tactics for medication treatment of youth depression (Hughes et al. 2007). For adolescent depression, the NIMH-funded multisite Treatment for Adolescents With Depression Study (TADS) (Treatment for Adolescents With Depression Study [TADS] Team 2003) compared fluoxetine, CBT, the combination, and placebo in 439 adolescents with major depressive disorder (MDD). Summary findings were that on the Child Depression Rating Scale, fluoxetine (with or without CBT) was superior to placebo in efficacy with an acceptable risk-benefit profile and that at week 12 of treatment, combined treatment and fluoxetine alone were equal in benefit and had greater benefit than CBT, which was not significantly different from placebo (TADS Team 2004). Rate of response with combined treatment was greater than that for CBT, but the results of all active treatments converged by 18 weeks (Kennard et al. 2009). Further analysis showed that combined treatment had an advantage over fluoxetine alone for mild to moderate depression but no significant advantage for moderate to severe depression.

The subsequent NIMH-funded six-site Treatment of Resistant Depression in Adolescents (TORDIA) study included 334 adolescents with MDD or dysthymia who had not responded to an adequate trial of an SSRI for at least 8 weeks. Subjects were randomly assigned to one of four conditions: switch to a different SSRI (predominantly citalopram) or to venlafaxine or addition of CBT to either of those medication switches. Adding CBT to either medication switch was more effective than a medication switch alone. There was no difference in efficacy between switch to another SSRI or venlafaxine, but venlafaxine produced more side effects (Brent et al. 2008). The initial trajectory by 6 weeks of treatment predicted whether the patient would remit, suggesting that clinicians should not wait longer than 6–8 weeks to switch or add treatments if the patient is not responding.

Even with evidence-based treatments, many youth remain impaired and vulnerable to relapse. Research is ongoing to find strategies to improve remission rate and reduce or delay relapses. Systematic research in youth is lacking, but for severe (especially if psychotic) depression unresponsive to adequate trials of pharmacotherapy, electroconvulsive therapy (ECT) may be considered. Transcranial magnetic stimulation appears to be useful in depressed adults, but there has been no controlled study in adolescents.

The use of antidepressants and mood stabilizers is discussed in Chapter 8.

It is extremely difficult to implement controlled trials in youth with bipolar disorder. Attempts have been made to extrapolate from research on adults, but the findings are not consistent. All of the medications have significant side effects (see Chapter 8). Drugs with current FDA indications for pediatric bipolar disorder/mania are lithium (age 12 years and older); the atypical antipsychotics aripiprazole, risperidone, and quetiapine (age 10 years and older); and olanzapine (age 13 years and older; consider other drugs first due to weight gain). Aripiprazole and lithium are also approved for prevention of recurrence of mania. Compared with adults, youth with mania have greater response to the atypical antipsychotics, but youth experience lower effect sizes with the mood stabilizers divalproex and lithium. In a direct comparison in youth with bipolar disorder, risperidone was faster and more effective than divalproex in acutely reducing symptoms of mania (Pavuluri et al. 2010). In contrast to the usual preference for monotherapy in pediatric psychopharmacology, combinations of medications are often needed for this disorder. Efficacy in bipolar depression remains elusive. Because of the risk of precipitating mania, antidepressants are generally not used in bipolar depression until treatment with a mood stabilizer is established. Family-focused treatment (FTT-A) has been shown to assist in reducing symptoms of depression in adolescents with bipolar disorder, when added to optimized pharmacotherapy (Miklowitz et al. 2008).

Children and adolescents who have seasonal affective disorder may respond to morning treatment with bright white light (Swedo et al. 1997).

■ ANXIETY DISORDERS

Phobias, PTSD, OCD, and panic disorder can begin in childhood or adolescence, but they are placed in the "adult" anxiety disorders section of DSM-IV-TR. (Separation anxiety disorder is covered in Chapter 4.)

Although fears and anxiety occur normally during development (see Table 5–5), anxiety disorders in children remain underrecognized and undertreated and can lead to lack of social competence, rejection or neglect by peers, academic underachievement, and eventual reduced occupational and social relationship functioning. In contrast to the disruptive behavior disorders, anxiety disorders often cause more distress in the child than in the parents and are thus considered "internalizing" disorders.

TABLE 5–5.　**Common normal fears**

Developmental stage	Feared object or situation
Birth to 6 months	Loss of physical support
	Loud noises
	Large rapidly approaching objects
7–12 months	Strangers
1–5 years	Loud noises
	Storms
	Animals
	The dark
	Separation from parents
3–5 years	Monsters
	Ghosts
6–12 years	Bodily injury/sickness
	Burglars
	Being sent to the principal
	Punishment
	Natural disasters
	Failure/rejection
12–18 years	Tests in school
	Low social competence
	Social evaluation
	Social embarrassment
	Psychological abnormality

Specific Phobia and Social Phobia (Social Anxiety Disorder)

Clinical Description

The DSM-IV-TR criteria for these disorders are largely the same in young people and adults, although cognitive immaturity may limit the child's recognition that fear is excessive or unreasonable, and under age 18 years a duration of 6 months is required for specific phobia. Transient developmentally appropriate fears (see Table 5–5) do not usually require treatment. Phobias are distinguished by their severity, irrationality, persistence, and functional impairment, usually secondary to avoidance of the feared object. Social phobia is a pervasive fear of social encounters and public performances where there is the possibility of negative evaluation by others.

Epidemiology

Many children with phobias are never seen in a clinical setting because parents and teachers rarely refer children with anxiety or excessive shyness for treatment. The prevalence of specific phobias in youth, averaged over studies, is 5% (Ollendick et al. 2002). Phobias are more common among girls and younger children. Social anxiety disorder is estimated to occur in 2%–5% of youth (March et al. 2007). However, lifetime prevalence in the general population may be as high as 16% (Lipsitz and Schneier 2000). While nonreferred youth with simple phobia generally have less comorbidity than do those with other anxiety disorders, the children who do present for treatment tend to be more symptomatic with regard to both anxiety and comorbidities.

Etiology

Contributions to the development of childhood anxiety include biological influences (e.g., heredity, behavioral inhibition/temperament, autonomic reactivity, and anxiety sensitivity) and environmental influences (e.g., insecure attachment style, overcontrolling/critical/anxious parenting style, peer and social problems, and negative/stressful life events) (Connolly and Suarez 2010). Interactions among these factors are complex.

Course and Prognosis

Specific phobias may begin at any time during development. Phobic symptoms may follow association of a stimulus with an unexpected panic attack or a traumatic event. Most simple phobias remit spontaneously, but some persist. Youth with natural environment-type phobias fare more poorly and are more difficult to treat than youth with animal-type phobias (Ollendick et al. 2010). Social phobia, which tends to start in adolescence, can result in impaired social and academic/occupational functioning due to school avoidance, social withdrawal, substance abuse, and difficulty with dating and intimacy. In one large sample of youth, stressful life events were a significant factor in the development of social anxiety (Aune and Stiles 2009). The disorder tends to persist into adulthood and is associated with professional underachievement, depression, generalized anxiety symptoms, constrained social functioning, and significant functional impairment.

Evaluation and Differential Diagnosis

Parents are often unaware of phobic symptoms or social anxiety in their children, so the clinical interview with the child is especially important. Younger children may express their phobic anxiety as crying, irritability, argumentativeness, tantrums, freezing, or clinging, rather than verbalizing it or explicitly avoiding the feared object or situation. Older youth may quietly avoid the feared stimulus or present with general irritability. A careful patient history aims to elucidate the feared stimulus, circumstances surrounding the development of the phobia, behavior in response to the phobic object or situation, anticipatory or avoidant behaviors, and any secondary gain. Observations of behavior may also be useful. A self-report questionnaire or clinician-administered measure designed for the specific presenting anxiety symptoms can be helpful to measure symptom severity or track treatment response, especially when symptoms are difficult to elicit by interview. Family assessment is also critical.

Differential diagnosis includes *panic disorder, agoraphobia, separation anxiety disorder, PTSD, OCD, learning disorders, mood and psychotic disorders, pervasive developmental disorder,* and *eating disorders* (fear of eating or of gaining weight) or *physical conditions.*

Treatment

Clinicians often integrate several approaches to treat phobic disorders. Cognitive-behavioral treatments are generally the treatment of choice for children with phobias because they are the best studied and the most efficient. The positive effects of CBT appear to generalize in this context, as seen in a recent study in which treatment of the targeted specific phobia led to improvement of comorbid specific phobias and other anxiety disorders (Ollendick et al. 2010). Effective behavioral treatment requires that the child has the skills and the opportunities to manage the problem situation in alternative ways. The therapist evaluates the child's skill set, teaches new skills when necessary, and works with the family (and school if appropriate) to eliminate inadvertent reinforcement of phobic behavior.

For specific phobias, CBT approaches developed for adults, such as systematic desensitization and exposure and response prevention (ERP) techniques, can be used in children, with strategies modified for developmental and cognitive levels. Systemic desensitization techniques (depending on specific phobia type) can include real life ("in vivo") exposure, narrative stories ("emotive imagery"), modeling of coping behavior, and contingency management using shaping, positive reinforcement, and extinction techniques (King et al. 2005).

For treatment of social phobia, CBT programs incorporating psychoeducation, exposure techniques (practicing feared situations with gradual exposures using fear hierarchies), and social skills training are used with youth and caregivers. Published resources are available to provide instruction and worksheets for role plays of naturalistic exposures, social skill development such as meeting new people, and nonverbal communication skills for youth with social anxiety (Chorpita 2007). Supplemental CBT strategies to facilitate exposures include cognitive restructuring, active ignoring, time-out procedures, and use of positive reinforcement (reward contingency plans). Cognitive restructuring techniques aim to reduce cognitive, emotional, and behavioral symptoms by specifically addressing maladaptive, distorted, self-defeating, or unrealistic thought patterns. By challenging these negative cognitions (thought patterns) associated with anxiety-producing situations (e.g., school exams or evaluative social settings), youth learn to generate more positive and realistic thoughts, thus improving related feelings and reinforcing mastery, competence, assertiveness, and healthy problem-solving abilities.

Medication trials often include multiple anxiety disorders. Placebo-controlled pharmacological treatment studies support the use of the SSRIs fluoxetine, fluvoxamine, sertraline, or paroxetine in the treatment of social phobia (generally with comorbidities of selective mutism, separation anxiety disorder, and/or generalized anxiety disorder) (see Chapter 8). Medication generally is reserved for cases in which severe symptoms interfere with psychotherapy or in which there is only a partial response to psychotherapy alone. For these disorders, tricyclic antidepressants (TCAs) have been replaced by SSRI medications, which have superior safety and tolerability. Benzodiazepines have potentially problematic adverse effects, are contraindicated in youth with a history of substance abuse, and have not shown efficacy in controlled trials; they are therefore not recommended other than possibly as an adjunct short-term treatment with SSRIs in severe cases.

The FDA has issued a "black box warning" for the use of any antidepressant medication, including SSRIs, in the pediatric population because of a small but significant increased risk of suicidal thoughts (compared to subjects on placebo). Pharmacological studies of pediatric anxiety disorder did not find an increased risk of suicidality (as opposed to pediatric depression, where this effect was seen), but careful monitoring is nonetheless essential when SSRIs are being used, with particular attention paid to mood, agitation, and suicidal thoughts or behaviors (Connolly and Suarez 2010).

Generalized Anxiety Disorder

Clinical Description

Children with generalized anxiety disorder (GAD) have pervasive worries for at least 6 months about a variety of areas (see Table 5–6).

The DSM-IV-TR criteria require only one accompanying symptom for children, whereas adults must have three.

The key feature of GAD is uncontrollable worry. It is important to clarify in an individual child that the excessive anxiety is actually *out of proportion* to the situation rather than an expectable reaction to a significant life stressor. Habit disturbances, such as nail biting, hair pulling, or thumb sucking, are common in youth with GAD. Somatic symptoms such as headache, upset stomach, or fatigue may result in parental requests for extensive medical evaluations.

Epidemiology

Transient symptoms of anxiety are common in typically developing children. However, full GAD occurs in 10% or more of children and adolescents, with an average age at onset of 8.5 years (Keeton et al. 2009). GAD is diagnosed twice as often in females as in males (Costello et al. 2004). Comorbidity among the anxiety and depressive disorders is common. Additionally, the results of a large study confirm that anxiety disorders frequently present with overlapping symptoms rather than as a single/focused disorder (Kendall et al. 2010). Many children with GAD never receive treatment.

Etiology

The multiple possible risk factors and their complex biological and psychological mechanisms and interactions are a focus of current research (Beesdo et al. 2009). Anxiety disorders are likely neurodevelopmental in their origins with genetic contributions, as are many other psychiatric disorders. This recognition is based on animal model research and human studies that have focused on critical developmental periods for specific neural circuits that mediate anxiety and appear to be sensitive to adverse events (Leonardo and Hen 2008). Researchers are honing in on the "gene by environment" interactions that highlight temporal and complex relationships between genetics and environment. Family genetic studies reveal important contributing factors (e.g., behaviorally inhibited temperament or information processing biases) and research on environmental factors

TABLE 5–6.	**DSM-IV-TR diagnostic criteria for generalized anxiety disorder (includes overanxious disorder of childhood)**

A. Excessive anxiety and worry (apprehensive expectation), occurring more days than not for at least 6 months, about a number of events or activities (such as work or school performance).

B. The person finds it difficult to control the worry.

C. The anxiety and worry are associated with three (or more) of the following six symptoms (with at least some symptoms present for more days than not for the past 6 months).   **Note:** Only one item is required in children.

  (1) restlessness or feeling keyed up or on edge
  (2) being easily fatigued
  (3) difficulty concentrating or mind going blank
  (4) irritability
  (5) muscle tension
  (6) sleep disturbance (difficulty falling or staying asleep, or restless unsatisfying sleep)

D. The focus of the anxiety and worry is not confined to features of an Axis I disorder, e.g., the anxiety or worry is not about having a panic attack (as in panic disorder), being embarrassed in public (as in social phobia), being contaminated (as in obsessive-compulsive disorder), being away from home or close relatives (as in separation anxiety disorder), gaining weight (as in anorexia nervosa), having multiple physical complaints (as in somatization disorder), or having a serious illness (as in hypochondriasis), and the anxiety and worry do not occur exclusively during posttraumatic stress disorder.

E. The anxiety, worry, or physical symptoms cause clinically significant distress or impairment in social, occupational, or other important areas of functioning.

F. The disturbance is not due to the direct physiological effects of a substance (e.g., a drug of abuse, a medication) or a general medical condition (e.g., hyperthyroidism) and does not occur exclusively during a mood disorder, a psychotic disorder, or a pervasive developmental disorder.

has implicated adverse life events, exposure to negative information, and modeling as important. Parent and child contributions to symptoms are presumed to be bidirectional, including an association between child anxiety and parental control (van der Bruggen et al. 2008). Children at risk of developing more severe anxiety symptoms are characterized by psychosocial adversity, inattention, low prosociality in school, and high levels of maternal discipline (Duchesne et al. 2010).

Course and Prognosis

Among lifetime cases of GAD, remission occurs spontaneously in as many as one-third of cases (Wittchen et al. 1994). Although many anxious children improve with or without treatment, most experience a chronic course with waxing and waning symptoms. GAD appears to have a worse prognosis and a lower remission rate than separation anxiety disorder. A childhood diagnosis of anxiety disorder is associated with an increased risk of heritability, symptom severity, impairment, and development of a range of disorders across the life span (Egger and Angold, 2006).

Evaluation and Differential Diagnosis

In general, children report their own anxiety symptoms more accurately than their parents do about them. Parents may either underreport because they are not aware of the child's symptoms or report an exaggerated degree of child anxiety, influenced by the parent's own heightened anxiety. Parents and children may actually be reporting different symptoms as "anxiety." Self-report instruments such as the Screen for Child Anxiety Related Emotional Disorders (SCARED) (Birmaher et al. 1997), with both child and parent scales, and the Multidimensional Anxiety Scale for Children (MASC) (March et al. 1997) can aid in assessment of anxiety symptoms. The Pediatric Anxiety Rating Scale (PARS) (Research Units on Pediatric Psychopharmacology Anxiety Study Group 2002) was developed to assess separation anxiety, social phobia, and generalized anxiety symptoms, particularly in treatment research.

Other anxiety disorders, such as *separation anxiety disorder, panic disorder, phobia,* and *adjustment disorder with anxiety,* and the *depressive disorders* should be considered in the differential diagnosis of GAD. Unlike children with *ADHD,* who are also restless and fidgety, children with GAD worry excessively (although the two disorders can be comorbid). Because children with GAD often have somatic symptoms, a wide variety of physical illnesses is in the differential diagnosis. Determining the extent of an appropriate medical workup for symptoms such as recurrent headache or abdominal pain can be difficult because children with documented physical etiologies also report anxiety and depression. *Medical disorders* that can mimic an anxiety disorder include substance withdrawal or intoxication, hyperthyroidism, pheochromocytoma, asthma, and medication side effects.

Treatment

CBT is the first-line psychotherapy approach for the treatment of anxiety disorders. The therapeutic alliance, parental ability to participate in treatment, and likelihood of completing therapeutic homework are important to consider when assessing for CBT suitability. CBT techniques used in the treatment of youth with GAD include relaxation exercises, cognitive restructuring, ERP, and problem-solving techniques in order to target the physical signs of anxiety and excessive worry. CBT can be provided in individual, family, group, or school-based settings.

SSRIs (particularly fluvoxamine, sertraline, and fluoxetine) have empirical support for treatment of GAD, although there is no evidence that a particular SSRI is more effective than another. The combination of CBT with sertraline offers additional benefit compared with either treatment alone, based on a large randomized controlled trial (Walkup et al. 2008). The use of medication requires close monitoring for possible side effects, and long-term use has not been well studied (Keeton et al. 2009). Current guidelines suggest maintenance medication treatment for approximately 1 year from symptom remission, with tapering and discontinuation during a low-stress time of year and attention to resuming medication if symptoms recur. The black box warning on SSRIs is discussed in other sections of this book. Although venlafaxine, TCAs, buspirone, and benzodiazepines have been suggested as alternative drugs, either as monotherapy or in combination with SSRIs, their safety and efficacy have not been established, due to limited or inconclusive research.

Referral of parents for treatment is often important, particularly if a parent also has an anxiety, mood, or other psychiatric disorder. The therapist should work with the parents to anticipate future developmental events that may lead to parental overprotectiveness or unrealistically high expectations for the child's performance.

Posttraumatic Stress Disorder

Clinical Description

PTSD involves specific, persistent emotional and behavioral symptoms following direct or observed exposure to a serious traumatic event that makes the individual feel intensely fearful, helpless, or terrified. Symptoms are organized into three broad categories: re-experiencing of the traumatic event, avoidance of reminders of the event and/or generalized emotional numbing, and increased arousal.

Although the DSM-IV-TR criteria for PTSD are essentially the same for all ages, the diagnosis of PTSD in youth is not straightforward. Many of the criteria are difficult to ascertain in children due to cognitive and emotional developmental immaturity (Terr 1991). Immediate effects of trauma can include fear of separation from parent(s), of death, and of further anxiety. Additional symptoms may develop regarding repetition of the experience, situations that involve separation or danger, or other reminders of the event. Children often withdraw from new experiences or develop various new fears. Perceptual distortions can occur, including tactile, olfactory, visual, and auditory misperceptions. Although children may accurately remember many details of the experience, sequencing or duration of events is often distorted. Some children become more distractible.

Children often reexperience the event in the form of nightmares, daydreams, or repetitive and potentially dangerous reenactment in symbolic play or in actual behavior (rather than in flashbacks). Despite obvious similarities between the reenactments and the original event, children can be unaware of the connection. Even very young children can demonstrate, through play or dreams, memories of traumatic events that they cannot describe verbally. The denial, repression, and psychic numbing that occur in many adults are not typically seen in children who experience a single traumatic event; however, their behavior may become disorganized.

Children often manifest increased arousal by sleep disturbances, which may add to functional impairment (Pynoos et al. 1987). They may have somatic symptoms, particularly headaches and stomachaches. Regression (behavior characteristic of a previous developmental stage) is common as is agitation or irritability. Children often feel guilty because they survived but others did not, or because they failed to save others. This guilt may be exacerbated by shame or children's normal cognitive egocentricity and magical thinking, which may contribute to a belief that they caused the event by thought or action. Child symptoms of constricted affect and diminished interest in activities may be elicited from interviews with parents, teachers, or caregivers.

Epidemiology

The general prevalence of PTSD among children and adolescents following either a single event or chronic repeated trauma is not known, and there is controversy about the diagnostic criteria, especially in young children. Early childhood experts have developed alternative criteria for use in infants, toddlers, and preschoolers (Scheeringa et al. 2003). In the general population, PTSD prevalence ranges from 1% to 14%. A study of 337 school-age children found that one-quarter of the children who were exposed to trauma met the criteria for PTSD (McCloskey and Walker 2000). In this study, death or illness of a loved one was the top risk factor for PTSD, and these children had a variety of other psychiatric comorbidity. Rates of both trauma exposure and PTSD are higher in girls than in boys.

Etiology

PTSD is relatively unique in the DSM-IV-TR because it requires an identifiable etiologic agent—the extreme traumatic event (American Psychiatric Association 2000). Knowledge of predisposing or protective factors in the development of PTSD in children exposed to trauma is limited. Children who have experienced multiple stressors, prior loss, disturbances in family functioning, or psychiatric comorbidity are vulnerable to more severe and prolonged symptoms, but a sufficiently severe stressor can produce the disorder in a person without any predisposition. The rate of PTSD increases with the degree of proximity to the traumatic event. Multiple risk factors have been identified for developing PTSD after a disaster, including media exposure, panic symptoms, delayed evacuation, sense of endangerment, and premorbid anxiety disorder (Cohen and Mannarino 2010).

PTSD likely involves a complicated interaction of neuroendocrine dysregulation with psychological and social factors. Neurodevelopmental factors have also been considered in the induction or maintenance of PTSD. Abuse or neglect of children may cause cognitive and developmental delays as well as increased arousal or withdrawal secondary to changes in brain physiology. Given the high degree of comorbidity with both internalizing and externalizing disorders, it is possible that trauma affects functioning in a more generalized manner.

Course and Prognosis

In addition to the initial trauma, disasters often result in loss of home, isolation from usual social supports, and loss of parents or other family members, which can exacerbate PTSD. Symptoms may be partially ameliorated by a stable, cohesive, and supportive family and safe environment. Whether a "natural recovery" occurs from PTSD is controversial.

Symptoms of anxiety (especially separation anxiety disorder) or depression may be prominent. Impulsivity, difficulty concentrating, and decreased motivation may interfere with school performance. Many traumatized children develop a chronic sense of pessimism and hopelessness about the future. For the subset of youth with persistent PTSD problems, prognosis is poor if untreated, with studies showing that PTSD in childhood is a significant risk factor for adult suicide attempts, major depression, dissociation, and impaired overall functioning (Warshaw et al. 1993). A history of sexual or physical abuse during childhood is associated with increased risk of lifetime psychopathology, particularly for women (MacMillan et al. 2001).

Evaluation and Differential Diagnosis

At the time of clinical presentation, a traumatic event may or may not be obvious. PTSD should be suspected in any child or adolescent who has had a significant change in behavior or emotional state. As with other childhood psychiatric assessments, multiple informants should be interviewed, as the child may have difficulty describing the symptoms, the caregivers may not be fully aware of the trauma or of the child's emotional reaction, and avoidance can lead to underreporting of symptoms. The developmental history may suggest increased vulnerability. Teacher observations regarding changes in school behavior or achievement can contribute to the evaluation. Consideration should be given to the child's developmental level and cognitive and expressive language skills when evaluating for symptoms. In addition, cultural factors, gender, and family issues can influence the manifestation of symptoms.

Given the increased interest in PTSD in youth, rating scales and structured interviews have been developed for both clinical and research assessment. A multidimensional approach to assessment of PTSD includes evaluation of cognitive, emotional, and behavioral symptoms; social and cognitive development; family and community factors; and overall functioning. Often, parents are also suffering from PTSD or other disorders, and prompt referral for their treatment is critical.

Comorbidity is common in PTSD and frequently includes mood, anxiety, and/or behavioral disorder diagnoses. PTSD is distinguished from *adjustment disorder* by the severity of the stressor and the distinctive symptoms, such as repetitive reexperiencing of the traumatic event. PTSD can mimic many other disorders such as *ADHD, ODD, panic disorder, social phobia, depression, substance abuse, bipolar illness, psychotic disorders,* or a variety of *physical conditions,* and thus requires a careful and sophisticated assessment for an accurate diagnosis.

Treatment

Established by Congress in 2000, the National Child Traumatic Stress Network (www.nctsn.org) serves as a resource for developing and disseminating evidence-based treatment and education in the area of trauma.

There are several available evidence-based psychotherapy treatment models for youth with PTSD symptoms, all of which share the following common components: they are developmentally and culturally sensitive, informed by the neurobiological impact of trauma on children, include parents/caretakers/families, and aim to reestablish safety and trust, address trauma reminders, and address significant areas of dysfunction (Cohen and Mannarino 2010). Clinicians match one of the evidence-based or evidence-informed treatments to the individual child, considering developmental level, treatment setting, acceptance by the family, type of trauma, and other individual factors. The model with the strongest empirical support is trauma-focused cognitive-behavioral therapy (TF-CBT). Cohen et al. (2005) described overarching treatment components as summarized by PRACTICE: Psychoeducation and Parenting skills, Relaxation, Affective modulation, Cognitive processing, Trauma narrative, In vivo mastery of trauma memories, Conjoint child-parent sessions, and Enhancing safety. A similar model for use in schools is CBITS (Cognitive-Behavioral Intervention for Trauma in Schools), which is TF-CBT adapted to group therapy during the school day with limited parental involvement. Another model with some empirical support is Child-Parent Psychotherapy (CPP), a relationship-based model designed to improve interactions between young children and parents. An individual trauma-focused CBT for single-episode traumas, called Cognitive-Based CBT, has been developed and studied. More specialized modalities include the Surviving Cancer Competently Intervention Program (SCCIP), the UCLA Trauma/Grief Program for Adolescents, and Trauma Systems Therapy (TST). There are additional treatments being developed to target "complex trauma"—namely, trauma with comorbidities including substance abuse. Web-based curricula have also been developed to enhance dissemination of evidence-based treatments.

Experts agree that treatment of PTSD in youth should start with psychotherapy (rather than pharmacotherapy) unless there is a compelling rationale to add medication, such as a comorbid diagnosis that requires medication, clear dangerousness requiring immediate medication, or severe symptoms that persist despite psychotherapy. If medication is used, the limited evidence suggests SSRIs, propranolol, or clonidine (Cohen and Mannarino 2010). Keeping in mind the established high placebo response in youth, observed symptom gains may not be due to the medication.

Obsessive-Compulsive Disorder

Clinical Description

The DSM-IV-TR criteria for OCD include recurrent and persistent thoughts (or impulses or images) and behaviors (or mental acts) that are acknowledged as unreasonable and are accompanied by distress. The child may have either obsessions (worries) or compulsions (rituals), although most patients have both. Because children may not recognize the senseless or excessive quality of OCD (specified as "with poor insight" in DSM-IV-TR), the requirement that the patient have insight into the nature of the disorder has been waived for youth.

Epidemiology

OCD is more common than clinical populations would suggest. Symptoms are poorly understood by and embarrassing to children and therefore often concealed, which delays assessment and diagnosis. The disorder is underrecognized and underdiagnosed. The prevalence of OCD in children and adolescents is thought to be 1%–2%, although rates as high as 4% have been reported. Mild or transient rituals, obsessions, or compulsions are common in the general population. At various stages of development, ritualistic behaviors and compulsions are normal. Examples are rigid bedtime routines; collecting, arranging, and storing of objects; and concerns about dirt and germs in preschool and early-school-age children (Leckman and Bloch 2008). Onset of OCD peaks in preadolescence and again in early adulthood (Geller et al. 1998). Boys tend to have earlier onset than girls; however, by adolescence gender distribution is likely equal (Swedo et al. 1989). Neither gender nor age at onset influences the number, specific type, or severity of OCD symptoms. Childhood OCD generally has a more favorable outcome than adult-onset OCD (Geller 2010).

Etiology

OCD is a model neuropsychiatric disorder. The "serotonin hypothesis" for the etiology of the disorder initially developed following the success of SSRIs in the treatment of OCD. Family studies indicate a genetic diathesis, with greater genetic loading in pediatric OCD compared with adult-onset OCD. Neuroimaging suggests abnormalities in connections between the basal ganglia and the cortex. A cortico-striatal-thalamic circuitry mechanism has been implicated that involves neurotransmitter systems such as glutamate, dopamine, and serotonin-containing neurons (Rosenberg and Keshavan 1998). The scarcity of a known family history of OCD in many cases raises speculation about environmental influences.

Geller et al. (2008) found that increased perinatal events among children with OCD were associated with earlier age at onset, increased symptom severity, and comorbidity with ADHD, chronic tic disorder, anxiety disorder, and major depressive disorder. Both comorbid anxiety and externalizing psychopathology are associated with increased symptom severity and impairment (Langley et al. 2010).

Although the existence of pediatric autoimmune neuropsychiatric disorders associated with streptococcus (PANDAS) has been controversial, there is some evidence supporting the hypothesis that group A beta-hemolytic streptococcus (GABHS) infection is linked to disease onset and clinical exacerbations in a subset of youth with OCD and/or tic disorders (Kurlan et al. 2008). On the other hand, a recent prospective study found that documented streptococcal infections were not associated with exacerbations of tic or obsessive-compulsive symptoms in children who met criteria for PANDAS, compared with children with Tourette's disorder and/or OCD who did not have a PANDAS history (Leckman et al. 2011).

Course and Prognosis

OCD in children (as in adults) appears to be a chronic condition, following a waxing and waning course. A recent outcomes study found that 41% of youth with OCD continued to have OCD 9 years later and 40% of the participants had an additional psychiatric diagnosis at follow-up (Micali et al. 2010). However, many youth will experience partial or full remission. The most commonly reported obsessions include contamination, sexual or somatic thoughts, and overly moralistic worries. The most commonly reported compulsions are washing, repeating, checking, and ordering (Geller et al. 1998).

Factors associated with a more severe course include very early age at onset, psychiatric comorbidities, poor initial treatment response, longer illness duration, and having a first-degree relative with OCD. Complications of OCD can include impairment in peer relations, adult intimacy, and employment, as well as physical sequelae such as dermatitis secondary to washing rituals.

OCD in children is usually accompanied by other psychiatric disorders. These can include anxiety and mood disorders, tics or Tourette's disorder, speech and developmental disorders, ADHD, disruptive behavior disorders, or other psychiatric disorders.

Evaluation and Differential Diagnosis

Children and adolescents are often secretive about obsessions and compulsions. Temper outbursts, academic struggles, or eating changes may be the presenting concerns until obsessions and compulsions are carefully elicited with specific questions to the child, parents, and teachers. Pathological rituals need to be distinguished from normal developmental childhood routines, and careful assessments of impairment are critical. The Children's Yale-Brown Obsessive Compulsive Scale (C-YBOCS; Scahill et al. 1997) is the gold standard assessment tool for use at initial diagnosis and in symptom monitoring during treatment. It provides a standardized inventory of symptoms and aids in assessing severity, subjective distress, impairment, internal resistance, and degree of control.

Alternative diagnoses include *phobic disorder, Tourette's disorder, anorexia and bulimia nervosa,* and *schizophrenia. Neurological conditions* can precipitate OCD symptoms. The usefulness of throat culture and streptococcal antibody titers in the absence of sore throat is controversial. *Complex tics* may be hard to distinguish from compulsions. Patients with *pervasive developmental disorder* can exhibit obsessive-compulsive symptoms. *Stimulant medication* can induce overfocused or perseverative behaviors, especially at higher doses.

Treatment

CBT is the first-line treatment for mild to moderate OCD in youth. Medication should be considered when OCD symptoms are severe, in the presence of comorbid disorder or family dysfunction, when the patient or family resists engaging in CBT, or when a skilled CBT clinician is not available. In the Pediatric OCD Treatment Study (POTS; March et al. 2004), CBT and medication treatment with sertraline were equally effective, and each was better than placebo treatment, although subsequent data analysis examining OCD with or without tics revealed somewhat different treatment outcomes. Combining CBT and medication yielded the greatest treatment response. Specific CBT techniques used in the POTS included psychoeducation, cognitive training (cognitive restructuring), mapping OCD, ERP, and relapse prevention/generalization training. CBT has been extended to group therapy and family-based approaches.

In addition to sertraline, the SSRIs paroxetine, fluoxetine, and fluvoxamine, and the tricyclic antidepressant clomipramine, have been shown to be effective in childhood OCD (Geller et al. 2003), although clomipramine is typically reserved for treatment-resistant cases due to its side-effect profile and interactions with other medications. If medication augmentation is required, the most common addition (extrapolating from research with adults) is an atypical antipsychotic, particularly if there are concurrent tic disorders, pervasive developmental disorder symptoms, or mood dysregulation.

A recent open trial of intensive family-based CBT in youth with OCD who were medication nonresponders or partial responders suggested that this specific CBT modality was beneficial in reducing OCD symptoms, impairment, depression, behavioral problems, and family accommodation to the symptoms (Storch et al. 2010). Advocacy groups such as the Obsessive Compulsive Foundation or Tourette's Syndrome Association can provide additional guidance for families. Supportive therapy can be helpful to address individual, social, school, or family issues.

Panic Disorder

Clinical Description

Panic disorder and agoraphobia are rare in children but somewhat more common in adolescents. DSM-IV-TR diagnostic criteria and physical symptom profile are the same as in adults. Family studies and retrospective reports note continuity between pediatric and adult presentations. In panic disorder there is a cycle whereby anxiety sensations lead to escalating anxiety, which escalates the sensations, and so on. Panic symptoms include both physiological and psychological features that occur spontaneously. In youth, cognitive immaturity may preclude some characteristic cognitions during an attack (fear of dying, going crazy, doing something uncontrolled). Panic attacks generally include shortness of breath, palpitations, chest pain, paresthesias, trembling, dizziness, tachycardia, sweating, and hyperventilation. Panic disorder can occur with or without agoraphobia.

Epidemiology

Prevalence rates of panic disorder in adolescents vary between 0.6% and 5% (Ollendick 1998), with age at onset typically in late adolescence and early adulthood (American Psychiatric Association 2000). However, panic symptoms are much more common, with prevalence in adolescents reported as high as 63% (Ollendick 1998). Panic disorder is more common in females than in males.

Etiology

Twin studies suggest genetic contributions. Modeling may also contribute. Offspring of parents with panic disorder are at high risk for anxiety disorders. A recent review of 24 studies examining panic disorder and cigarette smoking concluded that cigarette smoking tends to both precede the onset of panic and to promote panic (Cosci et al. 2010).

Course and Prognosis

The evolution of panic symptoms and the natural history of the disorder in children are not clear, but evidence supports chronicity (Biederman et al. 1997). Children with panic disorder and agoraphobia have high rates of other anxiety and mood disorders as well as ADHD (Biederman et al. 1997). Prepubertal onset may signal greater severity (Vitiello et al. 1990). Youth with the somatic symptoms of panic disorder are likely to first seek the help of a pediatrician or an emergency room. Panic attacks can begin at the onset of or during an episode of major depression or separation anxiety disorder.

Evaluation and Differential Diagnosis

Children can report current panic attacks, but parent report is helpful to verify duration and history. Self-monitoring techniques may be useful in children, as in adults. Panic disorder in children is likely underdiagnosed, with the symptoms often attributed to separation anxiety disorder, hyperventilation syndrome, or situational or "normal" anxiety. Panic can be distinguished from *separation anxiety disorder* by the lack of temporal association between initial symptom presentation and separation from a major attachment figure.

Treatment

Education is essential for patients, families, and school staff (if symptoms interfere with school functioning). If the cause of physical symptoms is unclear, consultation with the primary care physician is indicated. A recent randomized controlled trial found a CBT treatment (Panic Control Treatment for Adolescents; PCT-A) to be feasible and efficacious in a small group of adolescents followed for up to 6 months posttreatment (Pincus et al. 2010). CBT strategies that are used with panic disorder are aimed at the reduction of the fear of sensations that trigger the anxiety response. They include relaxation techniques, cognitive strategies, and exposure and response prevention, which can involve interoceptive exposure (gradual exposure to physical sensations by using exercises such as breath holding, running in place, or spinning to precipitate dizziness, shortness of breath, or sweating). SSRIs should be considered for panic symptoms that are persistent and/or impair functioning despite therapeutic interventions.

■ GENDER IDENTITY DISORDER

In normal development, the child establishes a *core gender identity* (the self-identification as a boy or a girl) by age 3–4 years. *Gender constancy* is achieved by age 5–6 years. *Gender role behavior* (cultural norms of mannerisms, gait, clothing, toys, play activities, and sex of playmates) is established as early as age 1 year and is set by age 6 years. In general, girls are permitted a great deal more latitude in gender role behavior. In nonclinical populations of boys, cross-gender behavior is rare after age 6 years.

Clinical Description

Boys with gender identity disorder (GID) (Table 5–7) display effeminate mannerisms, dress in female clothes (improvising if necessary), and avoid rough-and-tumble play. Girls refuse to wear skirts or dresses or to engage in culturally expected female play, such as dolls, dress up, or house (except as the father). The onset is typically before age 5 years. Parents often tolerate or even encourage cross-gender behavior early on but later become more concerned.

Epidemiology

There are no epidemiological data on the prevalence of true GID in children. More boys than girls come to clinical attention, perhaps because of greater cultural permissiveness regarding gender roles and behavior for females than for males. Cross-gender behavior of clinical significance, but not meeting full criteria for GID, is common in 5- to 12-year-old boys referred to a psychiatric clinic for various other emotional and behavioral symptoms (Pleak et al. 1989). These patients might fall into the category of GID not otherwise specified, comorbid with their primary diagnosis.

Etiology

Various biological, psychodynamic, and psychosocial causative factors for GID have been proposed. No genetic or hormonal factor has yet been identified, although some evidence suggests that gender identity is determined by prenatal hormones acting on the developing brain. Family characteristics, such as lack of appropriate gender role modeling; parental wish for opposite-sex child; parent who treats child

TABLE 5–7.	**DSM-IV-TR diagnostic criteria for gender identity disorder**

A. A strong and persistent cross-gender identification (not merely a desire for any perceived cultural advantages of being the other sex).

In children, the disturbance is manifested by four (or more) of the following:

(1) repeatedly stated desire to be, or insistence that he or she is, the other sex

(2) in boys, preference for cross-dressing or simulating female attire; in girls, insistence on wearing only stereotypical masculine clothing

(3) strong and persistent preferences for cross-sex roles in make-believe play or persistent fantasies of being the other sex

(4) intense desire to participate in the stereotypical games and pastimes of the other sex

(5) strong preference for playmates of the other sex

In adolescents and adults, the disturbance is manifested by symptoms such as a stated desire to be the other sex, frequent passing as the other sex, desire to live or be treated as the other sex, or the conviction that he or she has the typical feelings and reactions of the other sex.

B. Persistent discomfort with his or her sex or sense of inappropriateness in the gender role of that sex.

In children, the disturbance is manifested by any of the following: in boys, assertion that his penis or testes are disgusting or will disappear or assertion that it would be better not to have a penis, or aversion toward rough-and-tumble play and rejection of male stereotypical toys, games, and activities; in girls, rejection of urinating in a sitting position, assertion that she has or will grow a penis, or assertion that she does not want to grow breasts or menstruate, or marked aversion toward normative feminine clothing.

In adolescents and adults, the disturbance is manifested by symptoms such as preoccupation with getting rid of primary and secondary sex characteristics (e.g., request for hormones, surgery, or other procedures to physically alter sexual characteristics to simulate the other sex) or belief that he or she was born the wrong sex.

C. The disturbance is not concurrent with a physical intersex condition.

D. The disturbance causes clinically significant distress or impairment in social, occupational, or other important areas of functioning.

as opposite sex; same-sex parent who is absent, distant, or depressed; disturbance in mother–child relationship; mother who is dissatisfied with her own gender or gender role; and violence in the family, have been proposed as etiological factors in individual patients. However, many patients with GID do not have these factors, and many children exposed to these dynamics do not develop GID. Children raised by transsexual, lesbian, or gay parents show no evidence of confusion about gender identity or role behavior.

Course and Prognosis

Peer relationships are usually significantly impaired. Children generally have rigid gender role expectations and do not welcome a child who does not conform to these, although tomboys have somewhat more latitude than effeminate boys, who are teased and ostracized. Adolescents can be particularly cruel to peers who do not conform to conventional notions of gender role. The pervasive discomfort of the young patient with GID leads to low self-esteem and interferes with school performance.

As a group, patients with GID have levels of comorbid psychiatric disorders equal to those of other clinically referred patients, although some youngsters with GID have few symptoms of other disorders. Separation anxiety is common in boys with GID.

Follow-up studies of clinical populations show that some effeminate boys become transsexual adults and may have difficulty in social adaptation. A larger number of boys with gender-atypical characteristics develop a homosexual orientation in adulthood, which does not warrant a psychiatric diagnosis. Clinically referred girls with GID show a variety of gender and sexual orientations as adults, although nonreferred tomboys almost always develop more typically feminine interests at puberty. Treatment of GID appears to be more effective in childhood than in adolescence. For children who subsequently develop transsexualism as adolescents or adults, treatment is medically and psychiatrically complex.

Evaluation and Differential Diagnosis

Sensitive clinical evaluation is required. Older children or adolescents with GID learn from repeated negative feedback not to verbalize their wishes or beliefs about their gender and their anatomy. Children with GID must be differentiated from those who simply do not meet the gender role expectations of their families or their culture. Children with GID can be distinguished from tomboys or boys who have more studious or musical interests (rather than rough-and-tumble play and sports) by the rigidity of their avoidance of the expected gender role, their profound unhappiness with their physical gender, and their discomfort with or dislike of their sexual anatomy. Pediatric evaluation is indicated to rule out a *physical or hormonal abnormality* such as hermaphroditism, congenital adrenal hyperplasia, or androgen insensitivity syndrome.

Treatment

The best documented treatment of prepubertal GID is behavior modification. Changes in role behavior can lead to changes in gender identity, as well as improved self-esteem and decreased depression. Techniques include social reinforcement of gender-concordant behaviors, ignoring of cross-gender behaviors, reinforcement of play with appropriate toys, response cost (loss of points or privileges) for gender-inappropriate speech or play, modeling and shaping of skills the child does not have, and facilitation of positive peer experiences. Generalization is not automatic, and results are best if the program is conducted at home, in school, and at the clinic and several behaviors are addressed. Cognitive-behavioral self-monitoring of mannerisms also may be useful. More recently, some parents and clinicians have accepted the child's cross-gender identification and focused on making the environment more supportive to the child. Transgender adolescents have become less secretive in some settings.

Family therapy is often indicated, as is treatment of coexisting mood or conduct disorders. Parent counseling is always needed.

■ SLEEP DISORDERS

Evaluation of Sleep-Related Complaints

Nearly 25% of all children experience a sleep disorder at some time. The most common problems are sleep talking, nightmares, nighttime waking, difficulty falling asleep, enuresis, bruxism, sleep rocking, restless legs syndrome, and night terrors. Assessment of sleep disorders includes pediatric history and physical examination, particularly seeking evidence of obesity, enlarged tonsils, middle ear problems, a seizure disorder, allergies, asthma, and medication use. The evaluation of the airway includes tonsillar size, nasal airflow, and facial abnormalities. Abnormal physical findings in a child with a sleep continuity disorder are relatively infrequent, however.

A sleep history includes details of the patient's physical environment for sleeping and inquiries about whether the patient awakens screaming and confused, walks or talks while asleep, has frequent nightmares, has enuresis, grinds his or her teeth, has nighttime fears, snores, experiences restless legs or nocturnal leg jerks, and rocks or bangs his or her head at night. Sleep habits are reviewed and include the sleep environment, sleep schedules, and intake of caffeinated beverages. Children may resist bedtime or develop diurnal patterns that include difficulty awakening, daytime sleepiness, fatigue, and naps. A sleep log or diary is useful.

Developmental and psychiatric histories are necessary to assess possible psychiatric etiology or comorbidity. In addition, details of recent stressors, parental reactions to sleep-related problems, substance abuse (in older children or adolescents), and the effects of prior behavioral and pharmacological interventions are needed. When there is persistent nighttime waking or persistent sleep loss, or sleep apnea or nocturnal epilepsy is suspected, a sleep laboratory evaluation (polysomnography) may be indicated, including sleep electroencephalogram (EEG), eye movements, electromyogram, airflow, respiratory effort, electrocardiogram, and video monitoring. A sleep-deprived EEG is useful in the evaluation of possible seizures. A drug screen may be needed in adolescents. Sleep deprivation is particularly prevalent during adolescence, when late-night activities and early-morning academic schedules limit the available hours for sleep. Many adolescents tend toward delayed sleep-onset and awakening, making it difficult to obtain the required 9–10 hours of sleep per night.

Dyssomnias

Dyssomnias, including insomnia, narcolepsy, and breathing-related sleep disorder, are characterized by disturbance in the initiation or maintenance of sleep or by an excessive amount of daytime sleepiness.

Insomnia

Clinical description. Patients with insomnia have persistent difficulty initiating or maintaining sleep (compared with norms for age) that results in impaired functioning.

Epidemiology. Most infants sleep through the night (or at least do not fuss when they awaken) by age 6–9 months. Up to one-half of all infants, however, have irregular sleep patterns and occasional or persistent night wakening throughout the first year. A study of children without sleep disorders found that 21% of 18- to 23-month-olds awakened during the night. Of the 24- to 29-month-olds, 31% took more than 30 minutes to fall asleep on more than 3 nights per week. Children ages 30–36 months are most likely to have difficulty settling for the night (16%) and express fears of the dark (24%) (Crowell et al. 1987). At age 5 years, more than 20% of children surveyed continued to wake during the night and call out to their parents. Parental reinforcement may have contributed to this behavior, however. By school age, children are normally asleep for 95%–97% of the time they are in bed (Carskadon and Dement 1987).

Etiology. Sleep patterns in infants and toddlers may be affected by perinatal complications, colic, separation anxiety, the absence of a favorite transitional object, and parent–child interactions. The schedule of daytime naps for preschoolers can contribute to problems sleeping at night. Young children with sleep continuity disorders have a higher rate of family stressors, including parental absence because of employment, family illness, and maternal depression.

Chronic insomnia is much more frequent in children with psychiatric disorders. It is often related to behavior or habit problems in settling for the night (especially in the child with ADHD, ODD, or separation anxiety disorder) or may be a symptom of mood disorder, pervasive developmental disorder, or schizophrenia.

Insomnia may be secondary to the use of caffeine or prescribed or over-the-counter medication (e.g., phenobarbital, decongestants, or stimulants) or substance abuse. Patients suffering from physical discomfort may have difficulty staying asleep.

Treatment.   After any psychiatric or medical cause is addressed, in young children the first steps are to remove any factors that interfere with sleep and to enhance structure that encourages sleep (e.g., a bedtime routine, the use of a transitional object, or a night light for the child who is afraid of the dark). Behavior modification removes the secondary gain of parental attention at night and provides positive reinforcement for the child who stays quietly in his or her own room. Older children and adolescents may benefit from hypnosis or relaxation techniques. Consistency among all family members is critical to success.

In adolescents with insomnia, behavior therapy can disrupt the conditioned association between bedtime habits and anxiety regarding inability to sleep. Sleep hygiene is improved by using the bed only for sleeping, establishing a regular sleep schedule, avoiding naps, and removing all electronic media and communication devices from the bedroom.

Hypnotic medications are not recommended for chronic use. Many children respond to sedatives with paradoxical agitation. Melatonin may assist with circadian regulation and assist in falling asleep at bedtime.

Narcolepsy

Clinical description.   Narcolepsy is characterized by sudden, un-controllable attacks of rapid eye movement (REM) sleep during wakefulness. Features in children are similar to those seen in adults, including excessive daytime sleepiness, cataplexy, hypnagogic visual hallucinations, and sleep paralysis. Children and adolescents have variable presentations, with few experiencing all four symptoms simultaneously. The diagnosis is made by polysomnography.

Epidemiology.   The prevalence of narcolepsy in youth is 1 per 10,000.

Etiology.   Narcolepsy may have an autosomal dominant genetic transmission but with very low penetrance. Although a family history of narcolepsy can support the diagnosis, many cases have no evidence of family predisposition.

Course and prognosis.   Onset of narcolepsy is typically in late adolescence or early adulthood, although one-fifth of narcoleptic adults have an onset before puberty. Sleep attacks and cataplexy may interfere significantly with schoolwork and peer relationships. Behavioral and emotional changes can develop early in the clinical presentation.

Differential diagnosis.   The most likely alternative diagnosis to narcolepsy is the *normal* increase in daytime sleep and reports of sleepiness in adolescence. Truly excessive daytime sleep may be an *avoidance* mechanism, even in the classroom, or secondary to *insomnia, environmental interference with sleep,* or *sleep apnea.* Sleep-onset or waking hallucinations may be misidentified as symptoms of *psychosis,* and cataplexy or sleep attacks may be confused with a *seizure disorder* or *conversion disorder. Substance use* or *withdrawal* should also be suspected when sleep continuity is disrupted.

Treatment.   Treatment of narcolepsy begins with educating the patient and family members about the nature and course of the disorder. A regular sleep schedule with scheduled naps is helpful.

Stimulant drugs (methylphenidate, amphetamine) are used to reduce sleep attacks, particularly while the child is at school. Modafinil (Provigil) is a nonstimulant wakefulness-promoting agent that is approved for use in narcolepsy. Very low doses of REM suppressant medications, such as protriptyline or clomipramine, are useful treatments for cataplexy or hypnagogic hallucinations.

Breathing-Related Sleep Disorder (Sleep-Disordered Breathing)

Clinical description. Breathing-related sleep disorder is characterized by episodes of partial or complete upper airway obstruction and is part of a spectrum of disorders that includes primary snoring and upper airway resistance syndrome (usually due to adenotonsillar hypertrophy). Children may show behavior problems that typically present as inattention or excessive daytime sleepiness or activity. They are, however, less likely to have daytime somnolence than are adults. The preferred term is sleep-disordered breathing (SDB).

Epidemiology. The prevalence of sleep apnea is thought to be approximately 2% for children between ages 2 and 6 years. SDB is likely more common, and often is unrecognized. There is an increased risk during midadolescence, with symptoms that mirror the adult presentation. Prior to puberty, SDB is equally likely in males and females.

Etiology. SDB is caused by the loss of patency of the upper airway, caused by structural or neurological factors. With obstruction, respiratory efforts increase and greater muscle activity and arousal lead to relief of the obstruction. Medical causes of SDB include obesity, tonsillar hypertrophy, nocturnal asthma, lax upper airway structures, maxillofacial abnormalities, neuromuscular disease, Down syndrome, hypothyroidism, and dysfunction of central control of breathing.

Course and prognosis. The degree of adenotonsillar hypertrophy does not correlate with the severity of symptoms. Polysomnography is required to make the diagnosis. Children with sleep apnea may have medical complications, including pulmonary hypertension, systemic hypertension, right heart failure, failure to thrive, short stature, and enuresis. Greater awareness of the disorder has decreased the incidence of medical complications. Psychiatric and academic difficulties may include developmental delay, irritability, aggressiveness, distractibility, inattention, and hyperactivity.

Treatment.   The treatment of SDB is most often surgical, typically a tonsillectomy and adenoidectomy, which is curative in the majority of cases. Continuous positive airway pressure (CPAP) is an approved alternative.

Parasomnias

These disorders disrupt sleep with abnormalities of arousal, partial arousal, or sleep-stage transitions. The patient does not complain of insomnia or sleepiness. Parasomnias include nightmare disorder, sleep terror disorder, and sleepwalking disorder.

Nightmare Disorder

Clinical description.   Occasional normal frightening dreams occur during REM sleep, more commonly in the second half of the night. If the youngster awakens, he or she rapidly becomes oriented and alert, can recount the dream, and rapidly falls back to sleep. Frequency of nightmares waxes and wanes as the child develops. DSM-IV-TR criteria for nightmare disorder require "repeated" awakenings caused by nightmares with "significant distress" and "detailed recall." The child frequently cannot return to sleep and will ask to sleep with the parents.

Epidemiology.   Among children ages 3–5 years, 10%–50% have recurrent nightmares that disturb their parents. Symptoms typically begin during preschool years and decrease in frequency with age. Occasionally, the disorder persists into adulthood.

Etiology.   No psychiatric conditions are associated consistently with nightmare disorder in children. Nightmares tend to increase with stress, sleep deprivation, fatigue, and change in sleep environment.

Differential diagnosis.   Alternative diagnoses to nightmare disorder are *sleep terror disorder, narcolepsy, panic disorder, PTSD,* and *drug-induced nightmares* (e.g., as a result of prescribed medication or abuse of alcohol or drug).

Treatment.   Reassurance is generally the best approach. The child should not be pressured to describe the nightmare but should be given an opportunity to talk about his or her fears. Sleep schedules should be normalized and sleep time increased for patients suffering from sleep deprivation. Children and adolescents with more persistent problems may require anxiety reduction techniques, such as relaxation, imagery combined with systematic desensitization, and dream reorganization.

Sleep Terror Disorder (Pavor Nocturnus)

Clinical description.   Episodes of sleep terror disorder typically occur during the first third of the night, in Stage 3 and 4 delta (non-REM) sleep, and last 1–10 minutes. The child looks terrified, screams, and appears to be staring, with dilated pupils, sweating, rapid pulse, and hyperventilation. The child is agitated and confused and cannot be comforted. Subsequently, when alert, the child typically has no memory of the episode but may have brief recall of a feeling of terror or of dream fragments. The child rapidly returns to sleep when the episode is over and in the morning has no memory of the event. The parents are far more distressed than the child.

Epidemiology.   Sleep terror disorder is often seen in children ages 3–6 years, but isolated episodes are common throughout childhood. The estimated prevalence of the full disorder in children is 1%–6%, and it is more common in boys than in girls. A study of sleep habits in middle-class 1- to 3-year-olds found the 1-week prevalence of at least one episode to be 7% (Crowell et al. 1987).

Etiology.   Sleep terror disorder is considered to be developmental and is not caused by psychiatric disorder. Sleep terrors can be increased by sleep deprivation or anything that fragments sleep, including fever, illness, a full bladder, SDB, and certain medications. Patients (or parents) may experience symptoms due to cumulative sleep loss, if night terrors are frequent. Family history of sleep terror is common.

Course and prognosis.   Age at onset is typically between 4 and 12 years, with spontaneous resolution by adolescence. The number and frequency of episodes are highly variable. Consecutive episodes may be separated by days or weeks, but in rare instances they may occur on consecutive nights.

Differential diagnosis.   Simple *nightmares* or *nightmare disorder* usually occur in the latter half of the night. Those children remember the dream and show less physiological arousal and confusion than do those with sleep terror disorder. Other alternatives are *hypnagogic or hypnopompic hallucinations* or *epileptic seizures* during sleep with postical confusion. Occasionally, patients with *breathing-related sleep disorder* will awaken in a state of panic that resembles sleep terror disorder.

Treatment.   Parents should be educated about the disorder and reassured that the episodes do not indicate a psychiatric or neurological problem. The child's sleep schedule is monitored to provide a sufficient amount of time spent in bed. The patient's safety should be assured by erecting gates across stairs and locking doors and windows to prevent leaving the house. Waking the child before the usual time of the night terror may abort attacks. However, waking the child during the event should be avoided because it may exacerbate or prolong the episode. Medication is used only if the episodes are frequent, put the child in physical danger, severely disrupt the family, or interfere with daytime functioning. A low dose of imipramine or diazepam decreases delta sleep and may temporarily treat sleep terror disorder. However, when the medication is discontinued, delta sleep rebounds and the disorder may recur (Crowell et al. 1987). If SDB is diagnosed, surgery can relieve both SDB and night terrors.

Sleepwalking Disorder (Somnambulism)

Clinical description. Sleepwalking disorder is characterized by repeated episodes of arising from bed and engaging in motor activities while still asleep. Episodes, which last a few minutes to a half hour, typically occur 1–3 hours after the child falls asleep, during Stage 3 and 4 delta (non-REM) sleep. The child or adolescent arises quietly and engages in perseverative, stereotyped movements (such as picking at blankets), which may progress to walking and other complex behaviors. He or she is difficult to awaken, and coordination is poor. Although the child may be able to see, the risk of injury is high. Speech, when present, is usually incomprehensible. The youngster may awaken and be confused, may return to bed, or may lie down somewhere else and continue sleeping. Morning amnesia is typical. Occasionally, the patient engages in inappropriate behavior, such as urinating in the closet. Young children tend to walk toward a light or sound. Older children may wake in an agitated state with garbled speech and a tendency to recoil when touched.

Epidemiology. A longitudinal study of children and adolescents between ages 6 and 16 years found a 40% incidence of sleepwalking and a yearly prevalence of 6%–17%. Only 2%–3% had more than one episode per month. Sleepwalking continued for 5 years in 33% and for 10 years in 12% of the group.

Etiology. Likelihood of sleepwalking is increased when the child is overtired or under stress. Internal stimuli (e.g., urinary urgency, SDB, or restless legs syndrome) or external stimuli (e.g., noise) may precipitate an episode. Sleepwalking tends be familial. Of patients who sleepwalk, 10%–20% have first-degree relatives with the disorder.

Course and prognosis. The onset of sleepwalking is usually between ages 4 and 8 years, with the peak prevalence at age 12 years. Most cases remit spontaneously by age 15 years.

Differential diagnosis.   Diagnostic alternatives to sleepwalking disorder include nocturnal *seizures* and *waking and wandering*. During a *sleep terror,* children occasionally walk in an attempt to escape frightening stimuli. *Breathing-related sleep disorder* may also cause sudden confusion and agitation that will lead the patient to wander.

Treatment.   Parents should be guided to remove hazards in the environment. They may need to lock the child's door. Children should maintain regular sleep schedules. If sleepwalking is frequent or dangerous, a low dose of imipramine at bedtime may be used. Pharmacological treatments are limited because symptoms tend to return after the medication is discontinued.

■ ADJUSTMENT DISORDERS

Clinical Description

Adjustment disorder is characterized by the development of a dysfunctional reaction that occurs within 3 months of the onset of a stressor and that adversely affects functioning. An adjustment disorder may be diagnosed in a person with another mental disorder only if an identifiable stressor leads to the development of symptoms that are not characteristic of the original disorder. Adjustment disorders have six subtypes, classified by symptoms of depression, anxiety, and behavior (conduct).

Common stressors in childhood and adolescence include parental divorce, change in schools, physical illness, the birth of a sibling, parental unemployment, and abuse or neglect. Adolescents may be particularly vulnerable to disruptions in a relationship with a boyfriend or girlfriend.

Epidemiology

The prevalence of adjustment disorders in community samples of youth is between 2% and 8%. Populations with particularly severe stressors (i.e., surgical patients) have high rates of adjustment disorder. Children and adolescents usually have mixed presentations with symptoms that are not predominantly affective or behavioral.

Etiology

The adjustment disorder is presumed to be precipitated by the identified stressor. The child's reaction to the stressor rather than the characteristics of the stressor determine whether the diagnosis is present. Even in cases where the patient's emotional response to the stressor may be expected, if the symptom presentation is causing significant impairment, a diagnosis of adjustment disorder is made.

Course and Prognosis

Symptoms of adjustment disorder will typically remit when the stressor is removed or when a new level of adaptation is reached. By definition, if the disorder lasts for more than 6 months after the stressor or its consequences have stopped, then a different diagnosis is warranted. The prognosis depends on the severity and duration of the stressor and its meaning to the child; the vulnerability of the individual; and the response of the family, school, and peers to both the stressor and the young person's reaction. In general, the prognosis is assumed to be benign, although patients can present with active and passive suicidal behavior, substance abuse, and recurrent somatic complaints. Patients with adjustment disorder are more frequently admitted to medical emergency rooms and inpatient units than are control groups without psychiatric symptoms.

Follow-up of adolescents 5 years after receiving a clinical diagnosis of adjustment disorder found that 57% were well, although 23% of these patients had qualified for another psychiatric diagnosis during the intervening period. Research diagnoses at follow-up included schizophrenia, affective disorders, antisocial personality disorder, and substance abuse disorders. One patient committed suicide (Andreasen and Hoenk 1982).

Evaluation and Differential Diagnosis

The clinician should obtain reports from the child, parent, and teacher to identify stressors, rather than assuming that the first reported or obvious stressor is the crucial one. Other psychiatric diagnoses should be sought. Adjustment disorder is a residual category and should be used only if the patient's symptoms do not meet criteria for another DSM-IV-TR disorder. In the past, overuse of the diagnosis of adjustment disorder (in an effort to avoid "labeling" children) has often obscured another psychiatric diagnosis. Expectable reactions to the death of a loved one should be classified as *uncomplicated bereavement.* If functional impairment is not evident, or if the degree of emotional or behavioral reaction is considered "normal and expectable," then a V code, such as *relationship problem* or *phase of life problem,* should be used. If the primary reaction to a stressor is exacerbation of a pediatric disorder (e.g., asthma or diabetes), the appropriate diagnosis is *psychological factor affecting medical condition.* If the stressor is sudden and catastrophic or potentially so, *PTSD* or *acute stress disorder* should be diagnosed if the other criteria for those diagnoses are met.

Treatment

Crisis intervention and time-limited psychotherapy techniques may be useful for treatment of adjustment disorder. Cognitive therapy to improve coping skills and problem-solving abilities and to reduce dysfunctional thoughts and beliefs in reaction to the stressor may be beneficial. Environmental intervention may be indicated to remove or ameliorate the stressor and to mobilize family and community support systems. Explanations to parents and teachers of the child's or adolescent's reactions may reduce impairment and shorten the course of the disorder. Active treatment of these disorders may reduce subsequent morbidity. For example, if adjustment disorder with depressed mood is debilitating, the same treatments as for major depression may be indicated.

■ REFERENCES

American Psychiatric Association: Diagnostic and Statistical Manual of Mental Disorders, 4th Edition, Text Revision. Washington, DC, American Psychiatric Association, 2000

Andreasen NC, Hoenk PR: The predictive value of adjustment disorders: a follow-up study. Am J Psychiatry 139:584–590, 1982

Aune T, Stiles TC: The effects of depression and stressful life events on the development and maintenance of syndromal social anxiety: sex and age differences. J Clin Child Adolesc Psychol 38:501–512, 2009

Beesdo K, Knappe S, Pine DS: Anxiety and anxiety disorders in children and adolescents: developmental issues and implications for DSM-V. Psychiatr Clin North Am 32:483–524, 2009

Biederman J, Faraone SV, Marrs A, et al: Panic disorder and agoraphobia in consecutively referred children and adolescents. J Am Acad Child Adolesc Psychiatry 36:214–223, 1997

Birmaher B, Khetarpal S, Brent D, et al: The Screen for Child Anxiety Related Emotional Disorders (SCARED): scale construction and psychometric characteristics. J Am Acad Child Adolesc Psychiatry 36:545–553, 1997

Brent DA, Emslie G, Clarke G, et al: Switching to another SSRI or to venlafaxine with or without cognitive behavioral therapy for adolescents with SSRI-resistant depression: the TORDIA randomized controlled trial. JAMA 299:901–913, 2008

Carskadon MA, Dement WC: Daytime sleepiness: quantification of a behavioral state. Neurosci Biobehav Rev 11:307–317, 1987

Chorpita BF: Modular Cognitive-Behavioral Therapy for Childhood Anxiety Disorders. New York, Guilford, 2007

Cohen JA, Mannarino AP: Posttraumatic stress disorder, in Dulcan's Textbook of Child and Adolescent Psychiatry. Edited by Dulcan MK. Washington, DC, American Psychiatric Publishing, 2010, pp 339–348

Cohen JA, Mannarino AP, Knudsen K: Treating sexually abused children: one year follow-up of a randomized controlled trial. Child Abuse Negl 29:135–145, 2005

Connolly SD, Suarez LM: Generalized anxiety disorder, specific phobia, panic disorder, social phobia, and selective mutism, in Dulcan's Textbook of Child and Adolescent Psychiatry. Edited by Dulcan MK. Washington, DC, American Psychiatric Publishing, 2010, pp 299–323

Cosci F, Knuts IJ, Abrams K, et al: Cigarette smoking and panic: a critical review of the literature. J Clin Psychiatry 71:606–615, 2010

Costello EJ, Egger HL, Angold A: Developmental epidemiology of anxiety disorders, in Phobic and Anxiety Disorders in Children and Adolescents. Edited by Ollendick TH, March JS. New York, Oxford University Press, 2004, pp 334–380

Crowell J, Keener M, Ginsburg N, et al: Sleep habits in toddlers 18 to 36 months old. J Am Acad Child Adolesc Psychiatry 26:510–515, 1987

Dias PJ: Adolescent substance abuse assessment in the office. Pediatr Clin N Am 49:269–300, 2002

Duchesne S, Larose S, Vitaro F, et al: Trajectories of anxiety in a population sample of children: clarifying the role of children's behavioral characteristics and maternal parenting. Dev Psychopathol 22:361–373, 2010

Egger HL, Angold A: Common emotional and behavioral disorders in preschool children: presentation, nosology, and epidemiology. J Child Psychol Psychiatry 47:313–337, 2006

Geller B, Zimerman B, Williams M, et al: Phenomenology of prepubertal and early adolescent bipolar disorders: examples of elated mood, grandiose behaviors, decreased need for sleep, racing thoughts and hypersexuality. J Child Adolesc Psychopharmacol 12:3–9, 2002a

Geller B, Zimerman B, Williams M, et al: DSM-IV mania symptoms in a prepubertal and early adolescent bipolar disorder phenotype compared to attention-deficit hyperactive and normal controls. J Child Adolesc Psychopharmacol 12:11–25, 2002b

Geller DA: Obsessive-compulsive disorder, in Dulcan's Textbook of Child and Adolescent Psychiatry. Edited by Dulcan MK. Washington, DC, American Psychiatric Publishing, 2010, pp 349–363

Geller DA, Biederman J, Jones J, et al: Is juvenile obsessive compulsive disorder a developmental subtype of the disorder? A review of the pediatric literature. J Am Acad Child Adolesc Psychiatry 37:420–427, 1998

Geller DA, Biederman J, Stewart ES, et al: Which SSRI? A meta-analysis of pharmacotherapy trials in pediatric obsessive compulsive disorder. Am J Psychiatry 160:1919–1928, 2003

Geller DA, Wieland N, Carey K, et al: Perinatal factors affecting expression of obsessive compulsive disorder in children and adolescents. J Child Adolesc Psychopharmacol 18:373–379, 2008

Hayward C, Killen JD, Taylor CB: Panic attacks in young adolescents. Am J Psychiatry 146:1061–1062, 1989

Henggeler SW, Clingempeel WG, Brondino MJ, et al: Four-year follow-up of Multisystemic Therapy with substance-abusing and substance-dependent juvenile offenders. J Am Acad Child Adolesc Psychiatry 41:868–874, 2002

Hughes CW, Emslie GJ, Crismon ML, et al: Texas Children's Medication Algorithm Project: update from Texas Consensus Conference Panel on medication treatment of childhood major depressive disorder. J Am Acad Child Adolesc Psychiatry 46:667–686, 2007

Kandel DB: Stages in adolescent involvement in drug use. Science 190: 912–914, 1975

Keeton CP, Kolos AC, Walkup JT: Pediatric generalized anxiety disorder: epidemiology, diagnosis, and management. Paediatr Drugs 11:171–183, 2009

Kennard BD, Silva SG, Tonev S, et al: Remission and recovery in the Treatment for Adolescents with Depression Study (TADS): acute and long-term outcomes. J Am Acad Child Adolesc Psychiatry 48:186–195, 2009

Kendall PC, Compton SN, Walkup JT, et al: Clinical characteristics of anxiety disordered youth. J Anxiety Disord 24:360–365, 2010

King NJ, Muris P, Ollendick TH: Childhood fears and phobias: assessment and treatment. Child Adolesc Mental Health 10:50–56, 2005

Kovacs M: The Children's Depression Inventory (CDI). Psychopharmacol Bull 21:995–998, 1985

Kovacs M: The course of childhood-onset depressive disorders. Psychiatric Annals 26:326–330, 1996

Kurlan R, Johnson D, Kaplan EL, et al: Streptococcal infection and exacerbations of childhood tics and obsessive-compulsive symptoms: a prospective blinded cohort study. Pediatrics 121:1188–1197, 2008

Langley AK, Lewin AB, Berman RL, et al: Correlates of comorbid anxiety and externalizing disorders in childhood obsessive compulsive disorder. Eur Child Adolesc Psychiatry 19:637–645, 2010

Leckman JF, Bloch MH: A developmental and evolutionary perspective on obsessive-compulsive disorder: whence and whither compulsive hoarding? Am J Psychiatry 165:1229–1233, 2008

Leckman JF, King RA, Gilbert DL, et al: Streptococcal upper respiratory tract infections and exacerbations of tic and obsessive-compulsive symptoms: a prospective longitudinal study. J Am Acad Child Adolesc Psychiatry 50:108–118, 2011

LeGrange D, Crosby RD, Rathouz PJ, et al: A randomized controlled comparison of family based treatment and supportive psychotherapy for adolescent bulimia nervosa. Arch Gen Psychiatry 64:1049–1056, 2007

Leonardo ED, Hen R: Anxiety as a developmental disorder. Neuropsychopharmacology 33:134–140, 2008

Lewinsohn PM, Clarke GN, Seeley JR, et al: Major depression in community adolescents: age at onset, episode duration, and time to recurrence. J Am Acad Child Adolesc Psychiatry 33:809–818, 1994

Lewinsohn PM, Klein DN, Seeley JR: Bipolar disorders in a community sample of older adolescents: prevalence, phenomenology, comorbidity, and course. J Am Acad Child Adolesc Psychiatry 34:454–463, 1995

Lipsitz JD, Schneier FR: Social phobia, epidemiology and cost of illness. Pharmacoeconomics 18:23–32, 2000

Lock J, Agras WS, Bryson S, et al: A comparison of short-and long-term family therapy for adolescent anorexia nervosa. J Am Acad Child Adolesc Psychiatry 44:632–639, 2005

MacMillan HL, Fleming JE, Streiner DL, et al: Childhood abuse and lifetime psychopathology in a community sample. Am J Psychiatry 158:1878–1883, 2001

March JS, Parker JD, Sullivan K, et al: The Multidimensional Anxiety Scale for Children (MASC): factor structure, reliability, and validity. J Am Acad Child Adolesc Psychiatry 36:554–565, 1997

March JS, Foa EB, Gammon E, et al: Cognitive-behavior therapy, sertraline, and their combination for children and adolescents with obsessive-compulsive disorder: the Pediatric OCD Treatment Study (POTS) randomized controlled trial. JAMA 292:1969–1976, 2004

March JS, Entusah AR, Rynn M, et al: A randomized controlled trial of venlafaxine ER versus placebo in pediatric social anxiety disorder. Biol Psychiatry 62:1149–1154, 2007

McCloskey LA, Walker M: Posttraumatic stress in children exposed to family violence and single-event trauma. J Am Acad Child Adolesc Psychiatry 39:108–115, 2000

McKenna K, Gordon CT, Lenane M, et al: Looking for childhood-onset schizophrenia: the first 71 cases screened. J Am Acad Child Adolesc Psychiatry 33:636–644, 1994

Mehler P: Diagnosis and care of patients with anorexia nervosa in primary care settings. Ann Intern Med 134:1048–1059, 2001

Mellin LM, Irwin CE, Scully S: Prevalence of disordered eating in girls: a survey of middle-class children. J Am Diet Assoc 92:851–853, 1992

Micali N, Heyman I, Perez M, et al: Long-term outcomes of obsessive-compulsive disorder: follow-up of 142 children and adolescents. Br J Psychiatry 197:128–134, 2010

Miklowitz DJ, Axelson DA, Birmaher B, et al: Family focused treatment for adolescents with bipolar disorder: Results of a 2-year randomized trial. Arch Gen Psychiatry 65:1053–1061, 2008

Minuchin S, Rosman BL, Baker L: Psychosomatic Families: Anorexia Nervosa in Context. Cambridge, MA, Harvard University Press, 1978

Mufson L, Dorta KP, Wickramaratne P, et al: A randomized effectiveness trial of interpersonal psychotherapy for depressed adolescents. Arch Gen Psychiatry 61:577–584, 2004

Ollendick TH: Panic disorder in children and adolescents: new developments, new directions. J Clin Child Psychol 27:234–245, 1998

Ollendick TH, King NJ, Muris P: Fears and phobias in children: phenomenology, epidemiology, and aetiology. Child Adolescent Mental Health 7:98–106, 2002

Ollendick TH, Ost LG, Reuterskjold L, et al: Comorbidity in youth with specific phobias: impact of comorbidity on treatment outcome and the impact of treatment on comorbid disorders. Behav Res Ther 48:827–831, 2010

Palla B, Litt IF: Medical complications of eating disorders in adolescents. Pediatrics 81:613–623, 1988

Pavuluri M, Henry D, Findling R, et al: Double-blind randomized trial of risperidone versus divalproex in pediatric bipolar disorder. Bipolar Disorders 12:593–605, 2010

Pincus DB, May JE, Whitton SW, et al: Cognitive-behavioral treatment of panic disorder in adolescence. J Clin Child Adolesc Psychol 39:638–649, 2010

Pleak PR, Meyer-Bahlburg HF, O'Brien JD, et al: Cross-gender behavior and psychopathology in boy psychiatric outpatients. J Am Acad Child Adolesc Psychiatry 28:385–393, 1989

Pynoos RS, Frederick C, Nader K, et al: Life threat and posttraumatic stress in school-age children. Arch Gen Psychiatry 44:1057–1063, 1987

Research Units on Pediatric Psychopharmacology Anxiety Study Group: The Pediatric Anxiety Rating Scale (PARS): development and psychometric properties. J Am Acad Child Adolesc Psychiatry 41:1061–1069, 2002

Rosenberg DR, Keshavan MS: Toward a neurodevelopmental model of obsessive-compulsive disorder. Biol Psychiatry 43:623–640, 1998

Scahill L, Riddle MA, McSwiggin-Harden M, et al: Children's Yale Brown Obsessive-Compulsive Scale: reliability and validity. J Am Acad Child Adolesc Psychiatry 36:844–852, 1997

Scheeringa MS, Zeanah CH, Myers L, et al: New findings on alternative criteria for PTSD in preschool children. J Am Acad Child Adolesc Psychiatry 42:561–570, 2003

Schmidt U, Lee S, Beecham J, et al: A randomized controlled trial of family therapy and cognitive behavioral guided self-help for adolescents with bulimia nervosa and related conditions. Am J Psychiatry 164:591–598, 2007

Schwartz RH, Wirtz PW: Potential substance abuse: detection among adolescent patients: using the Drug and Alcohol Problem (DAP) Quick Screen, a 30-item questionnaire. Clin Pediatr (Phila) 29:38–43, 1990

Storch EA, Lehmkuhl HD, Ricketts E, et al: An open trial of intensive family based cognitive-behavioral therapy in youth with obsessive-compulsive disorder who are medication partial responders or nonresponders. J Clin Child Adolesc Psychol 39:260–268, 2010

Strober M, Carlson G: Bipolar illness in adolescents with major depression: clinical, genetic, and psychopharmacologic investigation. Arch Gen Psychiatry 39:549–555, 1982

Swedo SE, Rapoport JL, Leonard H, et al: Obsessive-compulsive disorder in children and adolescents: clinical phenomenology of 70 consecutive cases. Arch Gen Psychiatry 46:335–341, 1989

Swedo SE, Allen AJ, Glod CA, et al: A controlled trial of light therapy for the treatment of pediatric seasonal affective disorder. J Am Acad Child Adolesc Psychiatry 36:816–821, 1997

Tarter RE: Evaluation and treatment of adolescent substance abuse: a decision tree method. Am J Drug Alcohol Abuse 16:1–46, 1990

Terr LC: Childhood traumas: an outline and overview. Am J Psychiatry 148:10–20, 1991

Treatment of Adolescent Depression Study (TADS) Team: Treatment for Adolescents with Depression Study (TADS): rationale, design, and methods. J Am Acad Child Adolesc Psychiatry 42:531–542, 2003

Treatment of Adolescent Depression Study (TADS) Team: Fluoxetine, cognitive-behavioral therapy, and their combination for adolescents with depression: Treatment for Adolescents with Depression Study (TADS) randomized controlled trial. JAMA 292:807–820, 2004

van der Bruggen CO, Stams GJ, Bogels SM: Research review: the relation between child and parent anxiety and parental control: a meta-analytic review. J Child Psychol Psychiatry 49:1257–1279, 2008

Vitiello B, Behar D, Wolfson S, et al: Diagnosis of panic disorder in prepubertal children. J Am Acad Child Adolesc Psychiatry 29:782–784, 1990

Walkup JT, Albano AM, Piacentini J, et al: Cognitive-behavioral therapy, sertraline, or a combination in childhood anxiety. N Engl J Med 359:2753–2766, 2008

Warshaw MG, Fierman E, Pratt L, et al: Quality of life and dissociation in anxiety disordered patients with histories of trauma or PTSD. Am J Psychiatry 150:1512–1516, 1993

Weissman MM, Wolk S, Goldstein RB, et al: Depressed adolescents grown up. JAMA 281:1707–1713, 1999

Windle M, Windle RC: Depressive symptoms and cigarette smoking among middle adolescents: prospective associations and intrapersonal and interpersonal influences. J Consult Clin Psychol 69:215–226, 2001

Wittchen H-U, Zhao S, Kessler RC, et al.: DSM-III-R generalized anxiety disorder in the National Comorbidity Survey. Arch Gen Psychiatry 51:355–364, 1994

Wolk SI, Weissman MM: Suicidal behavior in depressed children grown up: preliminary results of a longitudinal study. Psychiatric Annals 26:331–335, 1996

■ ADDITIONAL READING

Eating Disorders

LeGrange D, Eddy KT, Herzog D: Anorexia nervosa and bulimia nervosa, in Dulcan's Textbook of Child and Adolescent Psychiatry. Edited by Dulcan MK. Washington, DC, American Psychiatric Publishing, 2010, pp 397–415

LeGrange D, Lock J: Treating Bulimia in Adolescents: A Family Based Approach. New York, Guilford, 2007

Lock J, LeGrange D, Agras WS, et al: Treatment Manual for Anorexia Nervosa: A Family Based Approach. New York, Guilford, 2001

Rosen DS and the Committee on Adolescence: Clinical report-Identification and management of eating disorders in children and adolescents. Pediatrics 126:1240–1253, 2010

Substance-Related Disorders

American Academy of Child and Adolescent Psychiatry: Practice parameter for the assessment and treatment of children and adolescents with substance use disorders. J Am Acad Child Adolesc Psychiatry 44:609–621, 2005

Bukstein OC, Deas D: Substance abuse and addictions, in Dulcan's Textbook of Child and Adolescent Psychiatry. Edited by Dulcan MK. Washington, DC, American Psychiatric Publishing, 2010, pp 241–258

Kaminer Y, Winters KC (eds): Clinical Manual of Adolescent Substance Abuse Treatment. Washington, DC, American Psychiatric Publishing, 2011

Nagy P: Motivational interviewing, in Dulcan's Textbook of Child and Adolescent Psychiatry. Edited by Dulcan MK. Washington, DC, American Psychiatric Publishing, 2010, pp 915–924

Schizophrenia

Kuniyoshi JS, McClellan JM: Early onset schizophrenia, in Dulcan's Textbook of Child and Adolescent Psychiatry. Edited by Dulcan MK. Washington, DC, American Psychiatric Publishing, 2010, pp 367–379

Mood Disorders

American Academy of Child and Adolescent Psychiatry: Practice parameter for the assessment and treatment of children and adolescents with bipolar disorder. J Am Acad Child Adolesc Psychiatry 46:107–125, 2007

American Academy of Child and Adolescent Psychiatry: Practice parameter for the assessment and treatment of children and adolescents with depressive disorders. J Am Acad Child Adolesc Psychiatry 46:1503–1526, 2007

Birmaher B, Brent D: Depression and dysthymia, in Dulcan's Textbook of Child and Adolescent Psychiatry. Edited by Dulcan MK. Washington, DC, American Psychiatric Publishing, 2010, pp 261–278

Carlson GA, Meyer SE: Bipolar disorder, in Dulcan's Textbook of Child and Adolescent Psychiatry. Edited by Dulcan MK. Washington, DC, American Psychiatric Publishing, 2010, pp 279–298

Friedberg RD, McClure JM: Clinical Practice of Cognitive Therapy With Children and Adolescents: The Nuts and Bolts. New York, Guilford, 2002

Mufson L, Dorta KP, Moreau D, et al: Interpersonal Psychotherapy for Depressed Adolescents, 2nd Edition. New York, Guilford, 2004

Anxiety Disorders

American Academy of Child and Adolescent Psychiatry: Practice parameter for the assessment and treatment of children and adolescents with anxiety disorders. J Am Acad Child Adolesc Psychiatry 46:267–283, 2007

American Academy of Child and Adolescent Psychiatry: Practice parameter for the assessment and treatment of children and adolescents with post-traumatic stress disorder. J Am Acad Child Adolesc Psychiatry 49:414–430, 2010

Gender Identity Disorder

Zucker KJ: Gender identity and sexual orientation, in Dulcan's Textbook of Child and Adolescent Psychiatry. Edited by Dulcan MK. Washington, DC, American Psychiatric Publishing, 2010, pp 543–552

Sleep Disorders

Ivanenko A (ed): Sleep and Psychiatric Disorders in Children and Adolescents. New York, Informa Healthcare, 2008

6

DEVELOPMENTAL DISORDERS

The pervasive developmental disorders (PDDs), including autistic disorder, and specific developmental disorders are coded on DSM-IV-TR (American Psychiatric Association 2000) Axis I. Mental retardation is the only developmental disorder now coded on Axis II.

■ MENTAL RETARDATION

Clinical Description

The DSM-IV-TR diagnosis of mental retardation requires low intelligence (IQ of approximately 70 or below), deficits in adaptive functioning, and onset prior to age 18 years. Experts in this field now prefer the term "intellectual disability." Adaptive skills include communication, self-care, home living, social skills, community resource use, self-direction, health and safety, functional academics, leisure, and work. Clinical features vary according to the degree of retardation (Table 6–1).

Epidemiology

Prevalence of mental retardation in the United States ranges from 1% to 3%, depending on the definition of adaptive functioning, and is highest among school-age children. All levels of severity of mental retardation are more common in males (overall, about 1.5:1). Mental retardation secondary to a specific etiology is as common in

TABLE 6–1. Clinical features of mental retardation				
	Mild	Moderate	Severe	Profound
IQ	50–55 to about 70	35–40 to 50–55	20–25 to 35–40	Below 20–25
Percentage of mentally retarded population	85	10	4	1
Predominant socioeconomic class	Low	Less low	Even distribution	Even distribution
Academic level achieved by adulthood	6th grade	2nd grade	Below 1st grade	Below 1st grade
Education	Educable	Trainable (self-care)	Simple skills	—
Residence	Community	Sheltered	Mostly living in highly structured and closely supervised settings	Mostly living in highly structured and closely supervised settings
Economic	Makes change	Makes small change	Can use coin machines	Dependent on others for money management
	Holds a job	Supportive employment or sheltered workshop	Can take notes to stores when shopping	
	Budget planning with effort or assistance	Usually able to manage pocket money		

upper as in lower socioeconomic groups. When the etiology is not known, however, lower socioeconomic groups predominate, and the degree of retardation is usually mild.

Comorbidity

Of all mentally retarded children and adolescents, 30%–70% also have a psychiatric disorder. This rate is significantly higher than in youngsters of normal intelligence, in part because neurobiological and psychosocial causes of mental retardation place the child at greater risk of psychiatric disorder. Almost every diagnostic category in psychiatry is represented.

The most common presentation is a constellation of symptoms that includes impulsivity, irritability, hyperactivity, short attention span, and language delay. The prevalence of attention-deficit/hyperactivity disorder (ADHD) in mentally retarded individuals is between 4% and 11%, a rate nearly identical to that in the general population. Symptoms of ADHD can be observed even in nonverbal children. In children with mental retardation, inattention may be a sign of inappropriate expectations rather than of a behavior disorder. Frustration may lead to aggressive temper outbursts.

Autism and other PDDs are far more likely to occur in children and adolescents with mental retardation than in nonretarded children. Both mental retardation and autism can be caused by congenital rubella syndrome, tuberous sclerosis complex, and phenylketonuria. Some symptoms seen in autism, including self-injurious behaviors, social isolation, and communication deficits, also may be found in persons with severe mental retardation. Autism is diagnosed when there is evidence of severe social impairment relative to the patient's developmental level. Stereotypic movements, including hand shaking or waving, body rocking, head banging, mouthing of objects, self-biting, picking at skin, or self-hitting, are among the more common psychiatric presentations in mentally retarded individuals, especially those with an IQ below 50. Pica, rumination, cluttering, stuttering, and other language and speech disorders occur at increased rates in association with mental retardation.

Depression can be a complication of mental retardation (e.g., in response to extra burdens, poor self-image, and social stigmatization) or simply a coincidence, and occurs at a rate similar to or higher than that in the general population. The disorder is probably underdiagnosed, because greater attention is paid to individuals who are aggressive than to those manifesting sadness or withdrawal. Depression in verbal, mildly mentally retarded individuals presents with the typical symptoms, although the patient's reports may be more concrete. The diagnosis in moderately or severely retarded youth, however, requires observation in several settings. Occasionally, depression is confirmed only by successful pharmacological or behavioral treatment. Rarely, individuals with mental retardation may have rapid-cycling bipolar mood disorders. Suicidal ideation and behavior may occur among mentally retarded individuals.

Twenty-five percent of youth with mental retardation have significant symptoms of anxiety. Diagnoses include generalized anxiety disorder, phobias, panic disorder, posttraumatic stress disorder, and obsessive-compulsive disorder. Fears of failing and loss of caregivers are among the environmental factors that increase the vulnerability of persons with mental retardation to anxiety disorders. Patients with mental retardation may not have the cognitive or verbal skills to describe specific cognitive or emotional symptoms, increasing the clinician's reliance on behavioral observation and report of caregivers.

Etiology

Mental retardation results from psychosocial, biological, and environmental factors. In 30%–40% of cases, despite rigorous medical investigations, the etiology is unknown. Birth complications, prematurity, and low birth weight are no longer viewed as significant sources of mental retardation, except in extreme cases.

Most mild retardation is idiopathic, associated with sociocultural or psychosocial disadvantage and familial. Intellectual and adaptive deficits are presumed to be determined by the interaction of a polygenic mechanism and social factors (Table 6–2).

TABLE 6–2.	Psychosocial causes of mental retardation
Poverty	Malnutrition
	Disease and infection
	Inadequate preventive care and medical treatment
	Sociocultural deprivation
Parental factors	Limited intelligence and education
	Psychiatric disorders
	Inadequate help-seeking behavior
	Lack of psychosocial stimulation
	Poor parenting skills
	Child abuse and neglect
Lack of community programs	Early identification and diagnosis
	Early intervention and infant stimulation
	Specialized education
	Vocational training and independent living

Moderate, severe, and profound retardation are less likely to be idiopathic. Mental retardation is associated with more than 200 recognized syndromes. Known biomedical etiologies are identified in 60%–90% of cases of severe or profound mental retardation (Table 6–3).

Down syndrome (triplication of chromosome 21), the most common genetic cause of intellectual disability, occurs in about 1 of 800 births. Fragile X syndrome is the most common inherited cause of mental retardation (1 in 4,000 males and 1 in 8,000 females). Characteristic physical stigmata (long face, prominent ears, prominent jaw, and macroorchidism [large testes]) are seen most clearly after puberty. Patients may have a high arched palate; hyperextensible finger joints; soft, velvetlike skin; and flat feet. A review of the medical history may reveal seizures, recurrent infections, hernias, strabismus, or scoliosis.

Among patients with fragile X syndrome, cognitive impairment ranges from learning disabilities with a normal IQ to profound retardation. In females (who are partially protected by having two X chromosomes), a "carrier" state is associated with

TABLE 6–3.	**Biological causes of mental retardation**
Genetic	Single gene defects—dominant
	Inborn errors of metabolism—recessive
	Chromosomal abnormalities (e.g., fragile X syndrome, trisomy 21 [Down syndrome])
	Polygenic inheritance
Prenatal	Maternal illness (e.g., diabetes, toxemia)
	Maternal infection passed to fetus (e.g., rubella, cytomegalovirus, toxoplasmosis, syphilis, herpes, HIV)
	Toxins (e.g., alcohol, tobacco, narcotics, lead, anticonvulsants)
	Brain malformations
	Extreme malnutrition
	Intrauterine growth retardation
Perinatal	Extreme prematurity
	Blood group incompatibility
	Brain trauma
	Cerebrovascular accident
Infancy or childhood	Brain infection (e.g., meningitis, encephalitis)
	Head trauma
	Neurological disease
	Brain tumor
	Hypothyroidism
	Radiation
	Lead intoxication
	Asphyxia
	Severe malnutrition

mild mental retardation or specific developmental disorders. Behavior problems are particularly prominent in males, with 70% meeting diagnostic criteria for ADHD. Anxiety disorders are common. In female fragile X patients, shyness and social anxiety with poor interpersonal rapport, poor eye contact, social isolation, social oddness, and in some cases selective mutism, are prevalent. The behavior can appear schizotypal in nature. Language and speech deficits include poor abstraction, immature syntax, unusual speech rhythm, expressive and receptive language deficits, and articulation problems. Neuropsychological deficits include perseveration, inattention, poor concentration, and mood lability. Social interactions may be impaired by odd communication patterns and mannerisms. Autism is diagnosed in approximately 20% of patients with fragile X syndrome; others have prominent features of pervasive developmental disorder not otherwise specified (PDD NOS) or avoidant personality disorder.

Course and Prognosis

The course of mental retardation can be influenced by active treatment. Medical care should address underlying conditions that can cause brain injury (e.g., shunting for hydrocephalus, diet for phenylketonuria). Associated medical conditions that compromise the child's functioning can be prevented or adequately managed. Such conditions include seizures, otitis media, injury secondary to self-abusive behavior, and deafness and congenital cataracts associated with Down syndrome. Adaptive functioning outcome is also influenced by environmental variables, including parental intelligence, psychological resilience, and material resources, as well as community resources and barriers.

More severe levels of mental retardation are diagnosed before the child is school age, particularly when associated with a known phenotype or syndrome. In moderate to mild retardation, diagnosis is uncommon before age 5 years, rises sharply in the early school years, and peaks in the later school years. Higher prevalence during the school years is usually attributed to the adaptive and intellectual demands of school (especially for social interaction and abstract thinking). At all levels of severity, the normal sequence of cognitive developmental stages occurs, but the rate of developmental progress is slow and there is a ceiling on ultimate achievement. Delays in speech and language development may limit ability to express negative affect, leading to impulsive anger and low frustration tolerance. Insufficient financial resources, inappropriate or inadequate educational programming, and prejudices of communities and health care personnel can result in a wide variety of developmental, social, and medical complications. Mental retardation is not necessarily a lifelong affliction. Proper training that addresses clinical needs and uses the patient's strengths can improve the level of functioning.

Evaluation and Differential Diagnosis

Intelligence is routinely measured by standardized tests (see Table 2–7 in Chapter 2). For very young children, the Bayley Scales of Infant Development or the Denver Developmental Screening Test may be used to estimate level of cognitive development.

Adaptive functioning may be judged by many means, including standardized instruments for assessing social maturity and adaptive skills. The Vineland Adaptive Behavior Scales (see Table 2–7) assess typical performance (not optimal ability) of the "daily activities required for personal and social sufficiency." The information obtained by a semistructured interview of a parent or caregiver yields a multidimensional measure of adaptive behaviors in five "domains": communication, daily living skills, socialization, motor skills, and maladaptive behaviors. Age-dependent expected competency scores of adaptive skills are established for children from infancy to age 18 years at different levels of mental retardation. The ABAS-II (Table 2–7) incorporates current guidelines of the American Association on Intellectual Disability and Developmental Disabilities.

Medical evaluation begins with a careful history that includes a review of familial disorders, neurophysiological insults, diseases with progressive deterioration, and seizure disorder. The physical examination should include a neurodevelopmental assessment of functional abilities and impairments and the presence of abnormal neurological signs. Laboratory investigations are particularly important when the mental retardation has no clear etiology. Brain imaging may identify lesions that are surgically correctable or at least explanatory. If seizures are suspected, an electroencephalogram (EEG) is indicated.

Mental retardation requires modifications in the standard psychiatric examination, according to the level of language and cognitive development. These patients suffer from multiple disabilities and medical disorders that affect mood and behavior. Clinical assessment must be comprehensive and based on the patient's presentation in multiple settings. Hyperactivity, aggression, sadness, lack of enthusiasm, excessive anxiety, and formal thought disorder are not primary features of mental retardation and should lead to a full psychiatric evaluation, as should a significant change in mood, behavior, sleep, appetite, or level of adaptive functioning.

The differential diagnosis of mental retardation includes *environmental deprivation, learning disorders, autism and other PDDs, communication disorders, borderline intellectual functioning,* and *severe visual or hearing impairment.*

Treatment

To address the multiple disabilities and complications associated with mental retardation, developmentally sensitive multimodal treatment is optimal. The psychiatrist should coordinate medical and psychiatric evaluations, parental guidance (support, education, behavior management, educational and environmental planning, long-term monitoring, and advocacy), and the standard therapies for concomitant psychiatric disorders. It is important to ensure the safety of the patient and those around him or her.

Behavior modification techniques such as removing inappropriate attention; changing deviant communication patterns (e.g., rewarding use of words or sign); consistently applying social, self-care, academic, and vocational expectations; and using environmental contingencies can reduce the frequency and severity of self-injury, stereotypies, pica, and asocial behavior. The behavioral program should be consistent and applied across settings, including home and school. Specialists may provide educational and developmental training to enhance speech and language; motor, cognitive, social, and occupational functioning; and adaptive skills such as toileting, dressing, grooming, and eating.

Developmentally oriented psychotherapeutic interventions may be effective to manage crises or to address long-term psychosocial goals. Therapy can focus on tangible objectives for the patient, including greater independence, recognizing and expressing emotion, dealing with the reactions of others, developing social skills, and handling personal and practical challenges. Group therapy for adolescents and young adults can be useful for social skills training. Family therapy can focus on learning about the disability, emphasizing the patient's strengths, reducing guilt and overprotection, and fostering greater independence.

Although no pharmacological treatments are available for mental retardation per se, the frequency of concurrent Axis I disorders may suggest the use of psychotropic medication. Treatment effects are often difficult to assess in developmentally disabled patients. Their impaired verbal skills may complicate the diagnostic process, measurement of efficacy, and detection of adverse effects. Heterogeneity among children with intellectual disability leads to variability in treatment effect. Youngsters with structural brain abnormalities often react differently to medications than do children with normal IQ, even when target symptoms are similar. Medications used for medical or neurological disorders associated with mental retardation may have problematic side effects and should be started at lower doses with more gradual increases.

Medications typically used for ADHD are effective in the treatment of symptoms of impulsivity, hyperactivity, and inattention in ADHD in children with intellectual disability, although effect size is less and side effects are more prominent. Few studies exist on the psychopharmacological treatment of depression in these patients, but selective serotonin reuptake inhibitors (SSRIs), such as fluoxetine (20–40 mg/day), may improve mood, energy level, interest, and motivation with minimal side effects. Cyclic mood disturbances have been treated successfully with lithium, although patients may experience cognitive dulling, gastrointestinal distress, tremor, fatigue, and a worsening of eczema. In these cases, carbamazepine or valproic acid is a reasonable alternative. Mentally retarded patients may present with aggression and self-destructive behavior that require prompt intervention and have led to the use of medications. A significant change in typical behavior warrants an investigation for a medical cause of discomfort. Or, these behaviors may be a symptom of a psychiatric disorder such as depression, bipolar disorder, or schizophrenia. Atypical antipsychotic agents have generally replaced typical neuroleptics because individuals with mental retardation are more susceptible to tardive dyskinesia and akathisia. Empirical support is greatest for risperidone, although weight gain and metabolic syndrome may be problematic (Aman et al. 2002). SSRIs or lithium may be successful in the treatment of aggression, stereotypies, self-injury, and compulsive behaviors.

■ PERVASIVE DEVELOPMENTAL DISORDERS

PDDs are divided into several categories that include autistic disorder, Asperger's disorder, and PDD NOS (to accommodate atypical or less severe cases). In these disorders, development is not merely delayed but also qualitatively atypical. PDD is not simply a collection of delays in specific skills or domains but implies broad disruption of functions.

Autistic Disorder

Clinical Description

The DSM-IV-TR criteria for autistic disorder (Table 6–4) focus on severe impairment, relative to chronological and mental age, with onset by age 3 years, in three key areas: social interaction, communication and play, and interests and activities. Autistic disorder has a wide spectrum of severity.

Social deficits are the most consistent and reliable indication of autism. Younger children fail to seek out peer interactions, whereas older individuals may express an interest in friendships and seek interpersonal experiences but lack the skills to initiate and maintain relationships. Persons with autism show persistent deficits in appreciating the feelings and thoughts of other people and in understand-

---

TABLE 6–4. **DSM-IV-TR diagnostic criteria for autistic disorder**

A. A total of six (or more) items from (1), (2), and (3), with at least two from (1), and one each from (2) and (3):

    (1) qualitative impairment in social interaction, as manifested by at least two of the following:

        (a) marked impairment in the use of multiple nonverbal behaviors such as eye-to-eye gaze, facial expression, body postures, and gestures to regulate social interaction

        (b) failure to develop peer relationships appropriate to developmental level

        (c) a lack of spontaneous seeking to share enjoyment, interests, or achievements with other people (e.g., by a lack of showing, bringing, or pointing out objects of interest)

        (d) lack of social or emotional reciprocity

    (2) qualitative impairments in communication as manifested by at least one of the following:

        (a) delay in, or total lack of, the development of spoken language (not accompanied by an attempt to compensate through alternative modes of communication such as gesture or mime)

        (b) in individuals with adequate speech, marked impairment in the ability to initiate or sustain a conversation with others

        (c) stereotyped and repetitive use of language or idiosyncratic language

        (d) lack of varied, spontaneous make-believe play or social imitative play appropriate to developmental level

    (3) restricted repetitive and stereotyped patterns of behavior, interests, and activities, as manifested by at least one of the following:

        (a) encompassing preoccupation with one or more stereotyped and restricted patterns of interest that is abnormal either in intensity or focus

        (b) apparently inflexible adherence to specific, nonfunctional routines or rituals

        (c) stereotyped and repetitive motor mannerisms (e.g., hand or finger flapping or twisting, or complex whole-body movements)

        (d) persistent preoccupation with parts of objects

TABLE 6–4.   **DSM-IV-TR diagnostic criteria for autistic disorder** *(continued)*

B.   Delays or abnormal functioning in at least one of the following areas, with onset prior to age 3 years: (1) social interaction, (2) language as used in social communication, or (3) symbolic or imaginative play.

C.   The disturbance is not better accounted for by Rett's disorder or childhood disintegrative disorder.

ing the process and nuances of social communication. They prefer solitary games and relate to others primarily as "objects" in their play.

Spoken language is either delayed or totally absent, with patients unable to initiate or sustain reciprocal conversation. Communication is characterized by echolalia, pronoun reversals, and idiosyncratic meanings. Phonological (sound production) and syntactic (grammar) functions may be relatively spared, with more significant impairments of verbal semantics (sociocultural meanings) and pragmatics (rules of interpersonal exchange) and nonverbal aspects of communication. Imaginative and symbolic functions (e.g., use of toys in play) may be dramatically impaired and play is characterized by rituals, stereotypies, motor mannerisms, and preoccupations with parts of objects.

Most individuals with autism have subnormal intelligence, but a few show significant improvements in measured IQ with time or treatment. Poor performance may be a result of the patient's lack of interest in taking tests. Approximately 50% of autistic patients are mentally retarded. Subtest results are often greatly scattered and inconsistent over time. The patient may have unusual or special capacities (savant skills) in music, drawing, arithmetic, or calendar calculation.

Epidemiology

Estimated prevalence of autism, based on DSM-IV-TR criteria, is 30–60 per 10,000. Broader autism spectrum disorders occur more frequently. There is a male predominance of 4–5 to 1. Increased prevalence estimates are likely due primarily to broader diagnostic criteria and increased awareness.

Etiology

Autism is a strongly genetic condition. The etiology of autism spectrum disorders involves multiple genes. The prevalence of autism in siblings is 4.5%. Monozygotic twins have a higher rate of concordance (60%–90%) than dizygotic twins, but it is not 100%, thus implicating early environmental biological insults as well. There is no evidence that psychosocial factors or parenting patterns cause autistic disorder.

A specific medical cause of autism can be identified in some individuals, most often in those with profound or severe mental retardation. Perhaps 5% have fragile X syndrome, and there is an association with tuberous sclerosis. Seizure disorders appear in 35%–50% of patients by age 20 years, more commonly in the presence of concurrent mental retardation. Brain-imaging studies demonstrate a wide range of abnormalities but no diagnostic pattern.

Various autoimmune disorders are overrepresented. Neurochemical studies are not, however, diagnostic. Despite considerable attention in the lay press, there is no evidence that links the mumps, measles, and rubella (MMR) vaccine or the vaccine preservative thimerosal to autism.

Course and Prognosis

Autistic disorder is often apparent in early infancy, and parents may seek a pediatric opinion during the first year. In some patients, the full disorder does not appear until after age 3 years. An initial period of seemingly normal development may be followed by developmental arrest or by regression with loss of previously developed abilities.

Children with autism usually make gradual but erratic improvement, particularly during the school-age years. Occasionally patients make rapid unexplained developmental progress. Medical illness and environmental stress may precipitate regression, which may include more compulsive and self-abusive behaviors, occasionally requiring pharmacological intervention. Adolescents may experience either continued development or behavioral deterioration. Seizure disorders are more likely to appear during adolescence.

Educational and supportive services have a marked beneficial effect. Even more severely autistic persons can learn some adaptive skills. For the less severely impaired, treatment may lead to social skills and adaptations that permit employment and independent or group home living. Predictors of good adaptive outcome include higher IQ, better language skills (especially the ability to communicate verbally by age 5 years), greater social skills, and later appearance of symptoms.

As adults, many autistic individuals continue to improve gradually but retain clinical evidence of residual organic brain damage. Depending on the severity of the autistic disorder, perhaps one-third are able to function independently as adults. Adults remain socially impaired, however, and often oppositional. Expressive and receptive language may appear normal, but deficits in social communication and empathy persist.

Evaluation

The evaluation of the child with suspected autistic disorder should be a collaborative process. Early developmental and medical histories are important. As part of the psychiatric evaluation, a workup of autistic disorder includes assessment of language, cognition, social skills, and adaptive functioning. Speech and language specialty testing can document abnormalities in abstract and pragmatic language, encoding of complex information, and attentional skills. Neurological examination is used to detect possible inborn metabolic, structural, or degenerative diseases or seizures. An EEG (for seizure disorder or developmental regression) and chromosome analysis may be advised. Audiological examination for possible deafness and examinations for other sensory deficits may be done. Patients with a tendency to mouth objects are at greater risk for lead intoxication. A psychologist experienced with these difficult youngsters must evaluate intellectual potential. Standardized diagnostic checklists (e.g., the Childhood Autism Rating Scale [CARS]) are based on clinical observation and parental recall of early behavior.

Examples of brief screening instruments that can be used by primary care physicians or nurses with very young children are the Checklist for Autism in Toddlers (CHAT), which includes parent interview and observations of the child (Scambler et al. 2001), and the M-CHAT, which includes only parent interview (available at http://www.firstsigns.org/downloads/m-chat.PDF). The "gold standard" instruments for autism diagnosis are the Autism Diagnostic Interview—Revised (ADI-R) and the Autism Diagnostic Observation Schedule (ADOS), developed by Lord and colleagues (these two instruments are available from Western Psychological Services; www.wpspublish.com).

Differential Diagnosis

Autism should be differentiated from other *PDDs*. *Rett's disorder* occurs predominantly in females and includes deceleration of head growth, marked mental retardation, hand-washing stereotypies, and loss of purposeful motor skills. *Asperger's disorder* does not cause delays in language development, cognitive development, age-appropriate self-help skills, or adaptive behavior. The child develops intense but unusual interests and lacks social skills. *Childhood disintegrative disorder* has a characteristic pattern of developmental regression beginning at age 2 years. Differential diagnosis also includes congenital *deafness* (but deaf children typically learn an alternative oral or sign language, lose their isolative behaviors, and develop expressive communication), congenital *blindness* (but blind children relate socially), *developmental expressive and receptive language disorders* (but these children are typically more sociable, communicate well in gestures, and do not have stereotypic and repetitive behavioral patterns), and juvenile-onset *schizophrenia* (distinguished by hallucinations, delusions, and thought disorder). Children with pure *mental retardation* have a more even pattern of delays and fewer abnormalities in behavior or social relatedness. The differential diagnosis is particularly difficult in children with severe to profound mental retardation. In very young children, *reactive attachment disorder* may be a consideration, but these cases are typically characterized by severe neglect. In *selective mutism* the patient is able to speak in some situations. *Degenerative neurological diseases* or *Landau-Kleffner syndrome* (acquired epileptic aphasia) may resemble PDD.

Children or adults with autistic disorder may have comorbid mood or anxiety disorders or symptoms of overactivity, inattention, and impulsivity (the diagnosis of ADHD is excluded in the presence of PDD).

Treatment

Patients fortunate enough to have early access to rigorous multimodal treatment show significant improvement. The milieu should be highly structured and should include special education, speech and language instruction, vocational training (for adolescents), and teaching of adaptive skills. Behavior therapy reduces unwanted symptoms; promotes speech, social interaction, and assertiveness; increases self-reliance and self-care skills; and facilitates exploration. Parent guidance is critical, both to provide education and to deal with emotional reactions such as guilt or denial. Parents can contribute to the child's learning of language and self-care and adaptive skills, arrange for special education and for adjunctive services, and make long-term plans for the child. Training in behavior management skills is essential for a tolerable home environment and for maximizing the child's potential.

Acute hospitalization or longer-term residential treatment may be needed. Long-term follow-up is required, including periodic reassessment for the possible appearance of seizures or mood or anxiety disorders.

Psychotropic medications may be used to ameliorate disruptive behavior or to treat coexisting psychiatric disorders. However, especially in nonverbal patients, physical discomfort as a cause for new or increased aggression or self-injurious behavior should be ruled out. Low doses of nonsedating antipsychotics, in conjunction with a highly structured treatment program, may help control behavioral symptoms, reduce excessive activity levels, and enhance the effect of behavior therapy. Controlled studies of atypical antipsychotics such as risperidone demonstrate clinical effectiveness with a relatively tolerable side-effect profile. The strongest evidence is for risperidone (McCracken et al. 2002) and aripiprazole (Owen et al. 2009) in reducing disruptive behavior and irritability (FDA-approved indications). Common side effects are sedation and weight gain. The risk of tardive dyskinesia may be higher in these patients because of the length of treatment and perhaps biological vulnerability.

Psychostimulant medication or atomoxetine may decrease symptoms of impulsivity, overactivity, and distractibility. SSRIs such as fluoxetine are sometimes effective in reducing obsessive-compulsive behaviors or depressive symptoms in adolescents with autism. Clomipramine decreases the frequency of some self-abusive behaviors. The α_2-adrenergic receptor agonist clonidine has been effective in double-blind reports examining behavioral control, but side effects can be problematic.

This chronic and often severe disorder can lead to parental desperation, unrealistic endorsements, and nonscientific pursuits of unconventional treatments. The field is plagued by unsubstantiated treatments that are at best ineffective and at worst divert time, energy, and resources from conventional treatments, or even have toxic effects (Herbert et al. 2002).

Asperger's Disorder

Asperger's disorder, an increasing focus of interest from parents and professionals, is characterized by deficits in social interaction and repetitive, restricted, and stereotyped behavior and interests without delay in cognitive or language development. To a large extent, it overlaps with high-functioning autism.

TABLE 6–5.	DSM-IV-TR specific developmental disorders
Learning disorders	Reading disorder
	Mathematics disorder
	Disorder of written expression
Motor skills disorder	Developmental coordination disorder
Communication disorders	Expressive language disorder
	Mixed receptive-expressive language disorder
	Phonological disorder
	Stuttering

■ SPECIFIC DEVELOPMENTAL DISORDERS

In each of the specific developmental disorders (Table 6–5), there is a discrepancy between potential and actual acquisition of skills and knowledge, although there is controversy regarding the emphasis on impairment relative to IQ.

Epidemiology

Estimated prevalence of each of the specific developmental disorders in elementary school–age children ranges from 2% to 15%. About 5% of all school children in the United States are classified as having a learning disorder. Comorbidity among developmental disorders and with psychiatric disorders is common.

Etiology

Lower socioeconomic classes are overrepresented in the specific developmental disorders. There is a male predominance of at least 2:1. Etiology may vary among the disorders, but is presumably related to cortical deficits secondary to organic damage, delayed maturation, or genetics. Frequent comorbidity among specific developmental disorders suggests that these impairments reflect multiple cerebral dysfunctions.

Genetic influence is substantial. Family histories in all subtypes of specific developmental disorder show an overrepresentation of reading, speech, and language disorders in the siblings and parents of affected children, although pedigrees are not consistent with a single mode of transmission. Monozygotic (MZ) and dizygotic (DZ) twin concordance approximates 85% and 50% for reading, 75% and 45% for language, and 70% and 50% for math (Plomin and Kovas 2005).

Learning Disorders

Clinical Description

Learning disorders are defined by delay in expected cognitive development in specific abilities. The child functions below age or grade level. Academic or adaptive impairment is required. The delay is not secondary to a sensory defect or known neurological disorder. Reading disorder, or dyslexia, has the most research.

Etiology

Maternal smoking during pregnancy, low birth weight, and prenatal and perinatal mishaps, in addition to strong genetic influence, appear to be associated with the appearance of developmental reading disorder.

Course and Prognosis

Learning disorders are frequently unrecognized and present instead as school refusal, oppositional defiant disorder, depression, or somatoform disorder. These patients are embarrassed by their academic difficulties, dislike school, and avoid schoolwork. Diagnoses are typically made in grade school. In later school years, problems involving organizational skills may remain, even if basic skills were well remediated. In college and graduate school, individuals may have difficulty learning foreign languages, writing efficiently, or reading fluently.

Axis I disorders are overrepresented in families of patients with learning disorders. Psychological and behavioral complications of learning disorder include low self-esteem, anxiety, demoralization, poor frustration tolerance, lack of enjoyment in learning, passivity or rigidity in new learning situations, truancy, delinquency, and school dropout. A strong relationship exists between reading disorder and ADHD; some of this is attributable to heredity. The interaction between conduct disorder and learning disorder is likely to be complex and multifactorial. Comorbid depression or anxiety disorders are relatively common.

Over time, mild cases may resolve through persistent remediation, practice, and compensation for deficits, but others retain specific learning deficits as adults. Often, secondary emotional and behavior problems persist beyond the duration or direct relevance of the developmental deficits. Young women with reading disabilities tend to bear children at younger ages, while young men are more likely to be unemployed. Adults may need to make accommodations in their lives and choice of career to cope with residual deficits.

Evaluation and Differential Diagnosis

When the clinician or therapist is working with a child with suspected learning disability, the first step is no longer to request that the school test the child's IQ and academic achievement, seeking a gap between them. The current approach (federally mandated) for schools is to assess the child's academic functioning compared with same-grade peers and his or her response to specific academic intervention designed to remediate functional deficits. In this "response to intervention" (RTI) approach, further evaluation does not occur unless the child does not improve. Section 504 of the Rehabilitation Act of 1973 (called "Section 504"), a federal antidiscrimination civil rights statute, may also be used to obtain accommodations in school.

Because of the high rate of comorbidity, evaluation of learning disorders includes assessment of the full range of abilities (specific academic skills, speech and language, and motor function), cognitive tests (including IQ), and observation of the child's behavior and quality of teaching in the classroom. Testing procedures must be sensitive to the ethnic and cultural background of the patient. Other possible causes of academic delays are poor teaching, cultural background, lack of fluency in English, and reduced school attendance. The clinician also evaluates the child for possible *mental retardation, ADHD, mood disorder* (causing low motivation), *anxiety disorder* (causing reduced attention), and other psychiatric and neurological disorders. Children with *communication disorders* may need tests that use nonverbal measures of intelligence to evaluate learning disorders. Sensory perception tests are needed to rule out impaired *vision* or *hearing*.

Treatment

Because a variety of specialists and teachers may be involved in the education of a child with multiple deficits, multidisciplinary communication is vital, particularly during school transitions. The Individuals with Disabilities Education Act (IDEA) mandates for all children with disabilities the right to a "free appropriate public education," including special education and related services designed to address their needs in the least restrictive context possible (see http://idea.ed.gov). In practice, remediation of only basic skills is funded, and deficits must be severe to qualify (e.g., 2 years behind expected level). An Individualized Education Program (IEP) is designed for each qualifying child, but the quality of evaluation and treatment services varies. Part-time resource rooms, full-time self-contained classrooms, and mainstream classrooms (with special-education consultants) provide the major part of special education. Specialized schools and residential treatment programs are rarely used due to scarcity and expense.

The IEP includes specific accommodations, including (depending on the type of disorder) use of a calculator or word processor; time-extended or oral tests; individual or small-group tutoring; or self-paced programmed texts or computerized self-instruction. Behavioral techniques are often used to improve motivation, emphasize success, foster enjoyment of new skills, reduce rigidity in learning, and promote application in new situations.

Parents of children with learning disorders should be included in educational planning. Supportive counseling may help them to avoid contributing to a climate of negativity and criticism and to adjust their child's and their own expectations to anticipate slower-than-standard learning but (unlike mental retardation) with no clear ceiling on educational achievement.

Individual psychotherapy may help reduce secondary psychological complications such as low self-esteem, temper tantrums, lack of assertiveness, and inflexibility. Medication treatment is not helpful for specific developmental disorders but may be for concurrent disorders.

Motor Skills Disorder: Developmental Coordination Disorder

In developmental coordination disorder, there is delayed learning of motor skills that is sufficient to cause functional impairment and is not caused by a known physical disorder. About 6% of children ages 5–11 years have significant impairments of gross or fine motor abilities. ADHD is commonly also present. Remediation is warranted to minimize sequelae such as scapegoating by peers, sports avoidance, academic difficulties (due to slow and illegible handwriting), and vocational impairment.

Communication Disorders

Clinical Description

Communication disorders are defined by delays in specific speech or language abilities that interfere with academic or adaptive functioning and that are not a result of PDD, mental retardation, sensory deficit, or structural or neurological disorder. There is a continuum of increasing severity of impairment from stuttering and phonological disorder, through expressive language disorder, to mixed receptive-expressive language disorder. In mixed receptive-expressive language disorder, both decoding (comprehension) and encoding (expression) are impaired, leading to more severe academic and social disruption than in expressive language disorder alone. A child may have more than one disorder, and multiple cortical deficits are usually observed, particularly in sensory information processing and temporal auditory processing. Nonverbal comprehension may be preserved or impaired to varying degrees, but attempted compensation through spontaneous use of gestural language or nonverbal communication is common.

Epidemiology

Speech and language disorders are evident in about 5% of the school-age population. Language disorders are more common in males and in children with psychiatric disorders, mental retardation, or hearing impairment.

Etiology

Many aspects of motor, sensory, and cognitive development must be intact for speech and language to develop normally. By age 5 years, children are expected to speak fluently and to comprehend speech. Adult articulation skills should be present by age 8 years. The range of normal functioning is broad, and development of language and speech skills continues for many years. Development of articulation and vocabulary is highly influenced by the child's environment. Verbal and nonverbal communication skills include word finding (access and retrieval of verbal information), word relationships (semantics), sentence formation (syntax), giving and receiving feedback, following conversational structure and flow, responding to the context, adapting to meanings and external events (pragmatics), responding to one's internal sense of events, and monitoring one's own communication (metalinguistic skills). The development of these skills is a formidable task to achieve in 5 years.

The etiology of deficits is often unknown, but there is strong evidence for the heritability of expressive language disorders, with and without articulation problems. Environmental factors also contribute and may include faulty speech models within the family and lack of stimulation of language. Hearing loss, even if mild, plays a significant role in the etiology of language and speech disorders. During the period of language development, fluctuating hearing capacity or degrees of hearing loss that are considered medically insignificant can diminish measured verbal IQ and academic performance. Even mild hearing loss (25–40 decibels) may delay development of articulation, expressive and receptive language, reading, and spelling.

Course and Prognosis

Relative deficits in articulation (speech sound production), expression (oral language production and use), and reception (comprehension) may be observable by age 2–3 years. Delays in speech and language frequently improve during development, so that early delays are not strongly predictive of subsequent psychiatric and learning disorders. Children with mixed receptive-expressive language disorder, however, have a poorer prognosis than those with expressive language disorder alone. Speech and language skills are eventually acquired in most cases, but other characteristics (concomitant psychiatric disorders, neuromotor problems, low IQ) may predict worse outcome.

Complications of speech and language disorders include progressive academic impairment, psychological distress, low self-esteem, anxiety regarding learning, and school dropout. These children may have difficulty maintaining a conversation or expanding on a topic. Problems in social interactions may lead to peer problems and overdependence on family members. When frustrated, the young child may have tantrums or the older child may refuse to speak.

About 50% of children with communication disorders have concomitant Axis I diagnoses, and another 20% have other developmental disorders, especially academic skills disorders (Cantwell and Baker 1987).

Evaluation and Differential Diagnosis

Multidisciplinary assessment is required to evaluate communication disorders. Specialized speech and language evaluation includes articulation, receptive skills (understanding single words, word combinations, and sentences), and expressive language skills (syntactic structures, vocabulary, and social appropriateness). The clinician may observe family characteristics and free speech between parents and child to assess social skills and nonverbal communication (vocalizations, gestures, and gazes). The clinician should obtain hearing acuity evaluation using audiometry or auditory evoked response (which does not require the child's cooperation) and evaluate auditory attention (losing flow of conversation, inability to hear in a crowd, distractibility), discrimination, and memory. Nonverbal measures of IQ (see Table 2–7) are used in cases of suspected language delay.

Differential diagnosis includes *autistic disorder, selective mutism, deafness, mental retardation, medical and neurological disorders,* and *acquired aphasia.* In adolescence, social awkwardness, resistance to change, and low frustration tolerance may approach the severity of autistic disorder, but youngsters with specific communication disorders have better social communication, empathic awareness, and abstraction than do those with autism.

Treatment

Hearing deficits should be addressed whenever possible. Social involvement, imitation, and imaginative play are encouraged to increase verbal, communicative, and symbolic skills. Referral to a speech-language pathologist is essential. Interventions should be maintained until symptoms improve. Once a child is "mainstreamed," speech and language therapy and supplemental academic supports may still be required. Psychiatric treatment of concurrent attentional, emotional, or behavior problems and educational management of academic skills disorders may be involved.

Stuttering

Clinical Description

Stuttering, a disruption of speech timing and fluency, is characterized by involuntary and irregular hesitations and blocking and prolongations, repetitions, interjections and substitutions of sounds, syllables, and words. The dysfluency typically worsens during periods of performance anxiety or communicative stress. The symptoms are often absent during singing, reading aloud, talking in unison, or talking to pets or inanimate objects. People who stutter are acutely aware of their symptoms and cannot readily improve their speech by slowing or by focusing attention on their speech rate or rhythm. The disorder compromises academic, occupational, and social functioning.

Epidemiology

The prevalence of stuttering is about 1% in children and slightly less in adolescents. The male-to-female ratio is approximately 3:1.

Etiology

Current etiological theories of stuttering include genetic, neurological, and behavioral factors, probably reflecting several etiological subtypes. Familial transmission is common, with the disorder appearing in about 20%–40% of first-degree relatives (especially males).

In rare cases, stutterlike dysfluency can be caused by psychotropic medications (e.g., antipsychotics, lithium, alprazolam).

No evidence indicates that anxiety or family dynamics *cause* stuttering, although anxiety and frustration secondary to stuttering may worsen the dysfluency.

Course and Prognosis

For toddlers, stuttering is usually a transient developmental symptom lasting less than 6 months, but 25% of patients with early onset of stuttering have persistent stuttering beyond age 12 years. Stuttering usually begins at ages 2–4 years but occasionally onsets at ages 5–7 years; it rarely starts during adolescence. Spontaneous improvement occurs in 50%–80% of patients. At the onset of illness, the child is usually unaware of the symptom. The disorder typically waxes and wanes during childhood.

Complications include fearful anticipation, eye blinking, involuntary tension of the jaw and face muscles, tics, and avoidance of problematic words and situations. Negative reactions by family and peers may affect self-image, social skills, and language development and lead to academic impairment, occupational problems, and social withdrawal.

Evaluation and Differential Diagnosis

Evaluation of stuttering includes a full developmental history and neurological and audiological examinations. Referral to a speech-language pathologist for evaluation is indicated in all cases. The clinician should assess the dysfluency in monologue, conversation, play, and mild stress conditions and observe parent–child interactions for communicative stress placed on the child (e.g., rapid questioning, interruptions, repeated corrections, frequent topic shifts). Behavioral assessment documents secondary restrictions in social interactions and activities.

Treatment

Speech therapy, conducted by speech-language specialists, involves intensive training of fluent speech skills, the fostering of self-esteem and social assertiveness, and the use of behavior therapy methods, such as modification of environmental and conversational factors that trigger stuttering, relaxation, role-playing, feedback, practice in speaking in different settings (reading aloud, choral reading, alone, in a group, in front of a classroom, on a telephone), and talking with different people (parents, relatives, friends, strangers). Education and counseling of family members are advised.

Psychotherapy generally is not indicated but might be considered for secondary symptoms or associated problems. Antianxiety drugs have minimal value.

■ REFERENCES

Aman MG, De Smedt G, Derivan A, et al: Double-blind, placebo-controlled study of risperidone for the treatment of disruptive behaviors in children with subaverage intelligence. Am J Psychiatry 159:1337–1346, 2002

American Psychiatric Association: Diagnostic and Statistical Manual of Mental Disorders, 4th Edition, Text Revision. Washington, DC, American Psychiatric Association, 2000

Cantwell DP, Baker L: Developmental Speech and Language Disorders. New York, Guilford, 1987

Herbert JD, Sharp IR, Gaudiano BA: Separating fact from fiction in the etiology and treatment of autism: a scientific review of the evidence. Scientific Review of Mental Health Practice 1:23–43, 2002

McCracken JT, McGough J, Shah B, et al; Research Units on Pediatric Psychopharmacology Autism Network: Risperidone in children with autism and serious behavioral problems. N Engl J Med 347:314–321, 2002

Owen R, Sikich L, Marcus RN, et al: Aripiprazole in the treatment of irritability in children and adolescents with autistic disorder. Pediatrics 124:1533–1540, 2009

Plomin R, Kovas Y: Generalist genes and learning disabilities. Psychol Bull 131:592–617, 2005

Scambler D, Rogers SJ, Wehner EA: Can the checklist for autism in toddlers differentiate young children with autism from those with developmental delays? J Am Acad Child Adolesc Psychiatry 40:1457–1463, 2001

■ ADDITIONAL READING

American Academy of Child and Adolescent Psychiatry: Practice parameters for the assessment and treatment of children and adolescents with language and learning disorders. J Am Acad Child Adolesc Psychiatry 37 (10 suppl):46S–62S, 1998

Cohen M: A Guide to Special Education Advocacy: What Parents, Clinicians and Advocates Need to Know. Philadelphia, Jessica Kingsley Publishers, 2009

Pierce K: Developmental disorders of learning, communication, and motor skills, in Dulcan's Textbook of Child and Adolescent Psychiatry. Edited by Dulcan MK. Washington, DC, American Psychiatric Publishing, 2010, pp 191–202

Tanguay PE: Autism spectrum disorders, in Dulcan's Textbook of Child and Adolescent Psychiatry. Edited by Dulcan MK. Washington, DC, American Psychiatric Publishing, 2010, pp 173–190

Toth K, King BH: Intellectual disability (mental retardation), in Dulcan's Textbook of Child and Adolescent Psychiatry. Edited by Dulcan MK. Washington, DC, American Psychiatric Publishing, 2010, pp 151–171

7

SPECIAL CLINICAL
CIRCUMSTANCES

This chapter covers a wide variety of situations and conditions that are not psychiatric diagnoses but in which psychiatric clinical skills may be useful or even required. Emergencies require expert assessment and prompt intervention. The effects of family transitions or adolescent pregnancy may become apparent in pediatric or school settings. Childhood obesity and physical illness raise psychological issues. The children of parents with psychiatric disorders are often ignored by systems of care designed for adults.

■ EMERGENCIES

Assessment and Triage

Emergencies present most often in psychiatric, pediatric, or general hospital emergency rooms, but they also occur in other psychiatric and pediatric settings and in schools (Table 7–1). The clinician rapidly assesses the potential for physical danger or acute psychiatric deterioration, evaluates support systems, may initiate treatment, and makes a disposition for further evaluation and treatment. In situations that are potentially dangerous to the youth or to others, a delay in intervention may result in acute exacerbation or increased resistance to treatment or actual harm.

An emergency evaluation must be brief and focused (Table 7–2). The clinician should talk with the child or adolescent and the relevant adults both alone and together. Important collateral informa-

---

TABLE 7–1. **Common psychiatric emergencies in children and adolescents**

Suicidal behavior, threats, or intent

Victim of physical abuse or severe neglect

Victim of sexual abuse or rape

Violent behavior or threats of violence

Delirium or other behavior or mental status changes secondary to medical illness or to prescribed medication

Nonpsychotic hallucinations in young children

    Night terrors

    Acute phobic hallucinations

Psychosis

Acute anxiety reactions, hyperventilation, panic attack

Acute school refusal

Fire setting

Running away

Substance abuse

Anorexia nervosa or bulimia nervosa

Conversion symptoms

---

tion can be gathered by telephone, from as many informants as possible (with appropriate consent). To ensure patient and staff safety and facilitate immediate intervention, the clinician must assess immediately for

- Medical illness or medication side effect
- Head trauma
- Intentional or accidental overdose
- Drug or alcohol intoxication or withdrawal
- Need for physical restraint or containment to prevent aggression or elopement
- Need to prevent a parent from removing the child from the emergency room or the child escaping
- Drugs or weapons carried by or available to the patient

A careful mental status examination is crucial in an emergency

TABLE 7–2.	Outline of emergency history
Demographics	Age Residence School and current grade Financial status Primary caregiver
Chief complaint	Who initiated the emergency visit? What happened? What did the patient intend to do? How was the patient discovered? How did the patient and others react?
Past suicide attempts and intent	Overdose of prescribed or over-the-counter medication Use of firearms Hanging Other self-injury Presence of alcohol or illicit drugs
History of present illness	Development of symptoms Intervention attempts and their results Involvement of social agencies
History of emotional or behavior problems	Depression Aggression Conduct disorder Drug or alcohol use Psychosis
Adaptive functioning with family, school, and peers	
Stressors in patient and family	
Abbreviated developmental history	Mental retardation Regression from previous level of functioning

TABLE 7–2.	Outline of emergency history *(continued)*
Family situation	Family living arrangements
	Other family or adults involved or who could be involved
	Adult stability, competence, relationship with the patient, attitude toward the patient and his or her problems
	Physical abuse, neglect, substance abuse
Family history of psychiatric illness or suicide	
History of medical illness and review of symptoms	

situation, with special focus on signs of psychosis, organicity, intoxication, suicidality, poor judgment, or impulsivity. Medical evaluation should be pursued as indicated (Table 7–3). The cause of a sudden change in behavior should be considered organic until proven otherwise. "Medical clearance" in the emergency room does not guarantee the absence of physical disorder as a cause of psychiatric symptoms.

TABLE 7–3.	Emergency medical evaluation

Physical and neurological examination
    Potential causes of organicity
    Evidence of drug ingestion
    Evidence of physical or sexual abuse
    Medical complications of an eating disorder

Laboratory tests according to clinical indications
    Follow-up findings on medical history and physical examination
    Pregnancy test
    Blood and urine drug screen
    Blood alcohol level
    Tests for sexually transmitted diseases

TABLE 7–4.	**Options for emergency dispositions**

Begin crisis intervention in emergency setting

Send home with outpatient referral or appointment to return to emergency room

Provide family members with information on outpatient referral or appointment to return to emergency room

Observe in the emergency room

Contact child welfare or protective services for placement outside the home in a shelter or foster home or for supervision in the home

If the patient is medically unstable, hospitalize in pediatric unit (may need constant observation) with psychiatric consultation

Partial hospitalization program (day hospital) or intensive outpatient program

Psychiatric hospitalization

Involve juvenile court

The clinician often has difficulty making a definitive DSM-IV-TR (American Psychiatric Association 2000) diagnosis in a single evaluation in an emergency setting, especially if collateral information is limited. Only a triage decision regarding further evaluation and treatment may be possible. Abbreviated feedback, education, and explanation are appropriate in the emergency setting. When the disposition or treatment is uncertain, the primary issue is safety (Table 7–4). The decision whether to hospitalize a young person is often determined by the ability of supervising adults to tolerate the young person's behavior or to ensure safety.

Suicide

Suicidal behavior is life threatening in all of its forms and should, therefore, be taken seriously regardless of age or circumstance. In pediatric patients, adults may assume that the intention of the youth's suicidal behavior is not serious and may not seek treatment. Very young children may lack the cognitive and physical skills to act on suicidal ideation, but a preoccupation with self-destructive behavior suggests significant psychiatric disturbance. Even the most blatant "gesture" can prove fatal, especially in a child whose assessment of physical danger may be immature and unrealistic. The need for accurate and prompt identification of suicidal behaviors is essential given the tendency for these symptoms to recur within days or weeks.

Epidemiology

The National Youth Risk Behavior Survey, conducted by the Centers for Disease Control and Prevention in 2009, found that 14% of high school students had in the past year "seriously considered attempting suicide," and more than 6% made a suicide attempt. In prepubertal children, the male-to-female ratio of completed suicide attempts is 3:1; a figure that increases to 5:1 in the 15- to 24-year age group. However, the prevalence of suicidal ideation and attempts is higher in females by a ratio of more than 2:1. Males choose more lethal methods to attempt suicide, including firearms and hanging, whereas females resort to overdose, carbon monoxide poisoning, and jumping. Suicide attempts using firearms are particularly lethal, especially when combined with substance use. The most common means are guns. In males, a history of suicidal behavior increases the risk of completed suicide. The association in females is not as strong. Gay, lesbian, and bisexual youth may be more likely to become suicidal because they are at risk for multiple risk factors, including depression, substance abuse, sexual victimization, rejection by family, and bullying by peers.

Course and Prognosis

Psychiatric symptoms are a risk factor for serious and recurrent suicidal behavior. Nearly all suicide victims have a psychiatric disorder, particularly mood disorder, in boys often comorbid with substance abuse and/or conduct problems. Unfortunately, only one-third of suicide attempters are ever referred to a mental health service. Additional risk factors include previous noncompliance with psychiatric treatment, social isolation, poor school performance, abuse and neglect, parental psychiatric illness, and family history of completed suicide. Medical illness increases suicide risk, especially epilepsy or central nervous system damage secondary to trauma, infection, or chemotherapy. Adolescent suicides are often preceded by stressful events, including the loss of a romantic relationship; reprimands in school or at home; or academic, family, or legal difficulties. Access to firearms increases risk.

Evaluation

When evaluating a youth after a suicide attempt, the clinician should obtain a detailed history of the circumstances preceding and following the attempt; symptoms of mood disorder, substance abuse, or impulsive behavior; wishes to die or to influence others at the time of the attempt; whether a friend or family member has committed suicide (looking for "contagion"); and coping skills and supports in the patient and family. Patients may present with a decline in social functioning characterized by isolation, legal problems, school suspensions, and running away from home. The seriousness of the attempt is determined by a consideration of lethality and intention. *Lethality* is a measure of the likelihood of death and is based on method, location, and the likelihood of being found. *Intention* is a description of what the patient wished to happen and is based on information provided by the patient and the interpretation by the clinician. Patients with a previous history of suicide attempts or who use methods other than ingestion and superficial cutting should be considered at highest risk. Assessment of risk factors for subsequent suicide attempts is essential (Table 7–5). Information should be collected from multiple sources including the patient, caregiver, school, and any other individual close to the patient.

Treatment

In determining disposition, safety is the first concern. A brief hospitalization may be useful to complete a more detailed assessment and begin treatment, even in youths who deny continuing suicidality.

TABLE 7–5.   **Risk factors for repeat suicide attempt**

Patient history

Verbalization or threats regarding suicide

Substance abuse

Poor impulse control

A recent loss or other severe stressor

Previous suicide attempt(s)

A friend or family member who has committed suicide

Exposure to recent news stories or movies about suicide

Poor social supports

Victim of physical or sexual abuse

Nature of the attempt

Accidental discovery (versus attempt in view of others or telling others immediately)

Careful plans to avoid discovery

Hanging or gunshot

Family

Wishes to be rid of child or adolescent

Does not take child's problems seriously

Overly angry and punitive

Depression or suicidality in family member

Unwilling or unable to provide support and supervision

Mental status examination

Depression

Hopelessness

Regret at being rescued

Belief that things would be better for self or others if dead

Wish to rejoin a dead loved one

Belief that death is temporary and pleasant

Unwillingness to promise to call before attempting suicide

Psychosis

Intoxication

Compliance with outpatient treatment recommendations may be improved if the therapist provides an appointment date and time and contacts the patient and family before the initial visit. Family involvement in treatment planning draws them into the therapy and educates them about psychiatric diagnoses, the lethality of the behavior, and the purposes of treatment. Caretakers should be told directly to lock away potentially lethal medications and to remove firearms from the home (or at least lock them securely, with ammunition stored and locked in a separate location). Although "no-suicide contracts" or "safety plans" do not eliminate risk, the discussion can provide insight into the thinking of both patient and caregivers. Warning signals, triggers, and potential youth coping strategies and external supports are identified.

Subsequent treatment includes treating primary psychiatric disorders, improving problem solving and stress reduction skills, and stabilizing the home and school environment. A model of dialectical behavior therapy has been developed for suicidal adolescents (Miller et al. 2007).

Child Maltreatment

In all psychiatric evaluations, the clinician should retain a high index of suspicion and collect information about the possibility of physical or sexual abuse. All states have laws requiring professionals who suspect child abuse to report it to the designated authorities. Mandated reporting is not confined to *confirmed* abuse. If evidence is sufficient to raise a serious question, the situation must be reported to prompt an official investigation. Clinicians acting in good faith are immune from liability for reporting, but legal penalties are assessed for failing to report. When the clinician suspects abuse, he or she should tell the parents that an investigation will ensue and that helpful services may be available from the child protection agency. Abusive parents are often frightened by their loss of control and remorseful for the injury to the child. They are overwhelmed by stressors and may be relieved to have aid in protecting the child. If the child is in immediate danger, he or she should be admitted to a pediatric service (by means of a court order, if necessary) until the investigation and determination of disposition are complete. In cases of significant abuse in which the parent is the suspected perpetrator or is unable to protect the child, the protective service agency should place the child in an emergency shelter or foster home. At times, security guards or police may be necessary to complete the disposition and keep the parent from absconding with an abused child.

Physical and Emotional Abuse and Neglect

Epidemiology.   After rising for several decades, reported rates of child and adolescent physical abuse and neglect have decreased since the early 1990s. Reported rates of emotional neglect are likely to be underestimates because child protection agencies are primarily concerned with the physical safety of children. There are no gender differences until adolescence, when females are more likely to be victims of physical abuse. Fatalities are more likely in younger populations, with more than 75% in children younger than 3 years. The National Child Abuse and Neglect Data System (NCANDS) reported more than 1,700 U.S. child fatalities in 2008. This figure is likely an underestimate, given the official tendency to report ambiguous deaths as accidental.

Clinical description and etiology.   Physical abuse is defined as injury or risk of injury to a child younger than age 18 years as a consequence of being hit with a hand or object or being kicked, shaken, thrown, burned, stabbed, or choked by a parent or parent substitute. Children who are threatened, verbally abused, or given harsh but nonphysical forms of punishment are considered to be emotionally abused. The most common abuser is the child's parent or guardian or the boyfriend of the child's mother. Risk factors for abuse include social isolation of parents, violence between parents, management of behavior problems with corporal punishment, inappropriate expectations for the child's developmental level, caretaker use of alcohol and drugs, and stressors on the family such as unemployment and overcrowding.

Neglect is more difficult to define than abuse, and clarification often requires a pediatric hospitalization with a comprehensive medical, psychiatric, and social evaluation. Neglect may be considered in five categories: 1) medical care neglect, 2) gross safety neglect (lack of supervision), 3) physical neglect (food and shelter), 4) emotional neglect, and 5) educational neglect (the latter two types are not recognized by all states). Emotional neglect applies when the patient is not given adequate attention and affection or is exposed to traumatic and inappropriate behaviors. Poverty contributes even more powerfully to neglect than to abuse. Many neglecting parents have never experienced or witnessed appropriate parenting. Some are mentally retarded, and others abuse drugs or alcohol or have mental illness.

Evaluation. Physicians should have a high index of suspicion for abuse when evaluating an injured child whose presentation is atypical. The history may yield clues such as delayed seeking of medical care, an explanation that does not fit the injury or the child's developmental level, and frequently changing stories. Injuries characteristic of abuse include, but are not limited to

- Multiple injuries in various stages of healing
- Bruises in the pattern of fingers or belts
- Burns, especially from cigarettes or scalding by water
- Spiral bone fractures
- Head and eye injuries
- Ruptured viscera

Evaluation of suspected abuse or neglect includes a complete physical examination (with radiological studies as indicated) and private interviews with the parents; the child (if old enough to talk) or adolescent; and other persons, such as siblings, babysitters, relatives, and neighbors. Youth may hide abuse because of fears that peers or family members will respond negatively (e.g., blame the victim). Although corporal punishment of children by parents (and, in many states, by teachers or principals) is still accepted by many cultural groups in the United States, any injury inflicted by a hard object or by burning, shaking, or throwing should be considered abuse, as should prolonged or severe spanking.

Effects.   Abused and neglected children are at risk for cognitive deficits, neurological impairment, blindness, physical disability, or even death. Psychological sequelae vary widely in severity and nature, commonly including low self-esteem, difficulty trusting others, impaired social relationships, increased impulsivity and irritability, anhedonia, aggression, poor school performance, and self-destructive activities including suicide and a variety of risk-taking behaviors. Posttraumatic stress disorder (PTSD), reactive attachment disorder, or symptoms of dissociation may ensue. Abuse victims may have depressive, anxiety, oppositional defiant, conduct, or attention-deficit/hyperactivity disorders or substance abuse.

Interventions.   The initial goal of treatment is to prevent the recurrence of abuse. Interventions include hotlines and self-help groups (organized by Parents Anonymous) that are useful for motivated but socially isolated parents who have difficulty controlling their angry responses toward their children.

Victims need interventions for abuse related symptoms, as well as psychiatric evaluation with multimodal treatment as indicated. Day hospital programs provide a safe and nurturing environment to begin abuse specific interventions. Group play therapy can encourage interaction with peers and avoid the solitary play that frequently develops in maltreated children.

Parents at high risk include teenagers, new parents, impoverished single parents, and individuals with histories of substance abuse or cognitive limitations. Perpetrators have high rates of depression, substance abuse, and antisocial behavior requiring assessment and treatment. Education in normal child development and principles of behavior management may be useful. Some parents need concrete assistance with housing, food, and medical care. Therapeutic and supportive services are often best provided in the home, because many families are both poorly motivated and insufficiently organized to make use of traditional outpatient services. Short-term placement of the child in foster care may be necessary while parents regroup and/or obtain psychiatric treatment. Child welfare agencies and family courts should be encouraged to determine rapidly whether parents can be rehabilitated and the children returned or whether proceedings should be initiated to terminate parental rights. Too often a child is placed in a succession of foster homes, punctuated by unsuccessful returns to the parents.

Sexual Abuse and Rape

Epidemiology. Approximately 120,000 cases of sexual abuse are substantiated by child welfare agencies each year. Although the reported incidence of sexual abuse and rape is increasing with mandatory reporting laws and heightened public awareness, it is still likely to be an underestimate. National surveys estimate about 5 children per 1,000 are sexually abused or assaulted in a year. Females are more likely to be victimized than males by 4–5:1. Most perpetrators are male and usually known to the victim. Although the offenders in most reported abuse cases are fathers or stepfathers, retrospective studies also identify uncles or brothers as frequent perpetrators. Extrafamilial and intrafamilial sexual abuse of boys is less frequently reported and prosecuted, even though the psychological consequences may be debilitating. Recent high-profile cases of sexual molestation of young males may bring more clinical, therapeutic, and legal attention to this problem.

Evaluation. Sexual abuse varies widely in degree of sexual contact; amount of physical or psychological coercion; single vs. repeated incidents; and whether the abuser is a member of the household, another person known to the child, or a stranger. The child may tell a parent, a friend, or a teacher, or there may be physical evidence such as prepubertal vaginal bleeding; recurrent urinary tract infections; inflammation, bruises, or lacerations of the genitals or anus; venereal disease; or pregnancy. Sudden onset of compulsive masturbation, precocious sexual knowledge or behaviors, oppositional behavior, fears, running away, depression, sleep disturbance, somatic symptoms, or decreased academic performance may raise suspicion.

Rape or sexual abuse by a stranger is usually reported by the victim immediately, although boys are less likely to acknowledge abuse because of a fear of retribution, a desire to appear self-reliant, and the social stigma against homosexual behavior. The child is often seen acutely in the emergency room. Sexual abuse by a relative or family friend is more difficult for children to report, is often discredited by the mother, and may result in a family crisis. In cases of father–daughter incest, the mother may suspect or be aware of the abuse, but fear of the father or a wish to "protect the family" prevents her from taking action. The mother may even tacitly encourage the abuse. In these families, a daughter takes on many aspects of the role of the mother and wife who is less available because of depression or physical illness.

The purposes of the initial evaluation are

- To determine whether abuse is likely to have occurred
- To ensure that the child is protected
- To establish the need for medical and psychological treatment

It is important that the evaluation itself does not further traumatize victims of sexual abuse. A team approach, in which health and mental health care professionals work together with the child protection agency and the legal system, avoids subjecting the child to repeated inquisitions. A complete physical examination is indicated, preferably by a pediatrician or pediatric gynecologist who has experience in evaluating abused children and who can carry out the procedures required for legal evidence. The clinician should interview (together and separately) the child, parents, and siblings. Questions about the specifics of the abuse are best saved for private interviews. For children who have difficulty verbalizing, the opportunity to draw or use puppets may be helpful. The use of anatomically correct dolls is controversial. If the alleged perpetrator is not a member of the immediate family, his or her interrogation is often best left to agency or legal officials. More complete evaluation of psychiatric and developmental status should be deferred for a subsequent interview.

Children rarely make false allegations of sexual abuse, except when prompted by a parent embroiled in a custody dispute, adolescent vindictiveness (e.g., to remove a disliked stepfather), or a wish to disguise the teenager's voluntary sexual activity. When false allegations are suspected, a child and adolescent psychiatrist with special expertise should be consulted.

Effects. Victims of sexual abuse are at increased risk of behavioral and emotional problems, and are overrepresented in clinical psychiatric settings. Rates of psychiatric disorders increase as the children approach school age, probably because they begin to recognize the deviant nature of the abuse. Victims report higher rates of major depression, anxiety disorders, conduct disorder, borderline personality disorder, antisocial personality disorder, paranoia, somatization, and bulimia. A history of sexual abuse increases the likelihood of attempted suicide 2- to 14-fold. Full or partial PTSD is common. Symptoms include fear, startle reactions, reenactment of the trauma, flashbacks, sleep disturbance, and depression. Children and adolescents who are victims of particularly severe or long-lasting abuse may experience dissociative reactions and conversion symptoms. The tendency to reenact the trauma may lead to sexual behavior problems. Among victims, risk factors for emotional and behavior problems include family disruption, economic hardship, preexisting psychiatric diagnosis, and scapegoating of the child for reporting the abuse. Psychological symptoms include suicidality, fears, sleep disorder, low self-esteem, sexual precocity or preoccupation, impaired social adjustment, and subsequent sexual dysfunction as an adult. Promiscuity or, in contrast, a phobic reaction with sexual inhibition may develop.

Medical sequelae include damage to the genitals or rectum, acquired immunodeficiency syndrome (AIDS), and other sexually transmitted diseases, which may lead to pelvic inflammatory disease and infertility.

Interventions. The child must be protected from both further sexual abuse and the effects of reporting it, especially if the perpetrator is the father or the mother's boyfriend. The child should return home only if the abuser has been removed from and does not have access to the home and if the mother can and will protect the child.

Research on treatment for sexually abused children and adolescents is limited. Sexual abuse is an experience rather than a disorder and the treatment targets symptoms and dynamics. Symptoms resulting from abuse vary based on developmental level, with children more likely to experience anxiety and sleep disorders and adolescents more likely to experiment with drugs and delinquent behavior. There is an empirically supported model of cognitive-behavioral therapy for sexual abuse–related PTSD symptoms in preschool-age children (Cohen et al. 2004).

Treatment interventions are "abuse-specific" and encourage the expression of abuse-related feelings, correct cognitive distortions regarding the abuse, teach prevention skills, and encourage support from other abuse victims. Specific symptoms may persist, however, and require targeted interventions that may include psychopharmacology. The therapist should select a treatment approach based on the characteristics of the child, the presence of psychiatric symptoms, and the family context. Intermittent treatment may be required for effects of abuse that may not appear for months or years. There is no evidence, however, that psychiatric treatment for asymptomatic victims of abuse will prevent future problems.

In incest cases, legal pressure may be required to initiate and maintain treatment of the perpetrator. Therapy models that aim at improving family functioning have not been particularly successful. Many parents (whether perpetrator or spouse) of sexually abused children have been abused themselves, making it difficult for them to deal with their child's situation. These parents may benefit from a support group for adult victims of childhood incest. If alcohol is a precipitating factor, successful treatment of the alcoholism markedly decreases the risk of recidivism.

Out-of-Control Behavior

When a child or an adolescent is brought to an emergency room because his or her behavior is out of control (Table 7–6), the clinician

TABLE 7–6.	Causes of out-of-control behavior in children and adolescents

Temper outbursts
    Attention-deficit/hyperactivity disorder
    Oppositional defiant disorder
    Conduct disorder
    Mental retardation
    Pervasive developmental disorder

Anxiety-provoked aggression
    Separation anxiety disorder
    Panic disorder
    Obsessive-compulsive disorder
    Acute phobic hallucinations (especially in children ages 2–6 years)

Organic delirium
    Medical illness
        Fever
        Electrolyte imbalance
        Central nervous system infection, tumor, trauma, or vascular accident
        Seizures
        Endocrine or autoimmune disorder
        Hypoxia
        Metabolic disorder
    Adverse reaction to prescribed or over-the-counter medication
    Toxic ingestion
    Reaction to illicit substance
        Acute intoxication or toxic reaction
        Flashback
        Withdrawal
        Psychotic reaction to chronic drug use

Schizophrenia

Mania

Abuse or neglect
    Posttraumatic stress disorder

must first use whatever physical means are necessary to ensure the safety of the patient, family, and staff.

Evaluation

If a patient has been aggressive, it is important to determine whether a person or object actually has been harmed or only threatened verbally or with gestures. Detailed description of the aggressive behavior includes: precipitants, warning signs, evidence of an altered mental state, actual damage, need for physical restraint, repetitive behaviors, lethality (including access to firearms), solitary vs. group action, and response to any previous treatment. Cultural factors may affect both the precipitant and the response.

The mental status examination includes an assessment of current anger or violent intent, organic cognitive impairment, paranoia, delusions or hallucinations, and impulsivity.

Patients with mental retardation, neurological disorders, or delayed expressive and receptive language are more likely to communicate distress through aggression. The older and larger the youngster, the more seriously aggression must be taken. If attention-deficit/hyperactivity disorder, conduct disorder, psychosis, mental retardation, or drug abuse cause impulsivity and impaired judgment, a more restrictive environment may be needed.

Children and adolescents with a history of escalating violence and pervasive hostility are most problematic. Occasionally youth will show little guilt or remorse for their actions. The risk of aggressive behavior is increased by neuropsychological dysfunction and exposure to violence and/or physical abuse. Witnessed violence between caregivers may have a greater emotional effect than actual victimization of the child. In such instances, parents model the choice of aggression as a solution to problems. Family assessment is important because relationships among all family members are affected by violence.

Treatment

In the acute situation, medication is sometimes considered, although children have usually calmed and rarely require medication in the emergency room. Special caution in pharmacotherapy is needed if a medical disorder or drug ingestion is suspected. If necessary, acutely psychotic adolescents can be given an antipsychotic agent (see Chapter 8). Particular attention should be paid to the safe and appropriate use of seclusion and restraint, if needed. The indications are risk of harm to self or others and the failure of less restrictive interventions to control the patient's behavior.

In considering disposition from the emergency room, the clinician must consider the safety of vulnerable persons in the home (e.g., a baby) and the ability of the adults to supervise. Even if the behavior resolves quickly in the emergency room, these youngsters often have multiple social, psychological, academic, and behavior problems that require psychiatric follow-up. The courts and child protective services are frequently involved in disposition planning.

After safety is ensured, the goal of treatment is to address the underlying cause of out-of-control behavior. Psychiatric hospitalization is not effective in the treatment of severe conduct disorders, placing more emphasis on partial hospitalization, residential treatment, therapeutic school placement, and comprehensive home-based treatment programs. The success of outpatient therapy depends on the patient's and family's cognitive abilities and motivation, the severity of antisocial behavior, and use of a systems/ecological approach. Cognitive-behavioral programs like anger management training encourage greater individual control. Social skills training increases alternatives to aggression, if the environmental contingencies can be managed to encourage their use. Family and, when necessary, the legal system should be involved and actively support the treatment process.

■ FAMILY TRANSITIONS

A substantial number of children spend some part of their life with just one parent, whether due to single motherhood, separation, divorce, or death of a parent. Children in single-parent households typically have more responsibility, not only for chores but also for management, decision making, baby sitting for younger siblings, and emotional support of the parent. As a result, these children may be more independent, competent, and responsible than other children but at the expense of having less freedom, more worries, and less closeness with peers. The parent–child relationship can suffer when children resent the additional responsibility.

Divorce

Effects

Divorce affects nearly all aspects of a child's life but does not have inevitable long-term negative consequences. It is a process that begins with marital strain and discord (that may last for years), is punctuated by the marital separation, and leads to dramatic changes in family life. To the child, divorce reflects the failure of a relationship that was to serve as a model of love and commitment. A conflict-ridden intact family is, however, more detrimental to children than a stable one-parent home. In fact, marital discord is a more important risk factor for child maladjustment than actual divorce or conflict following divorce (Buehler et al. 1998). High-intensity marital conflict during childhood is associated with attachment difficulties, externalizing and internalizing symptoms in childhood, and psychological disorders as young adults. Parental violence is even more detrimental to children's adjustment than verbal conflict. Rates of child abuse and sibling violence are increased in violent compared with nonviolent high-conflict marriages. Protective factors that have been identified for children in high-conflict marriages include a positive relationship with a caregiver and supportive siblings. In addition, for teenagers, peer relationships and a positive self-concept appear to be helpful. Another influence on the impact of high-conflict parental relationships is the manner in which parents settle their disputes. Unresolved or chronic discord is associated with more difficulties for children. Parental conflict in which each parent criticizes the other to the child and attempts to gain the child's alliance is particularly damaging, whether in an intact family or after divorce. Intense parental conflict may also reflect psychiatric symptoms in one or both adults. Children and adolescents commonly blame themselves for the divorce, view themselves as potential saviors, and harbor fantasies that their parents will reunite.

Reactions to parental divorce may vary with the age and developmental level of the child and the time since divorce. Infants may react with irritability and sleep and feeding difficulties. Children ages 2–6 years commonly experience separation anxiety and behavioral regression such as clinging or loss of toilet training. Children ages 5–9 years may be anxious, sad, and preoccupied with loss of their intact family and separation from their fathers (or sometimes their mothers), whatever the nature of the prior relationship. Slightly older children may feel shame and anger or complain of somatic symptoms, but have somewhat better coping mechanisms to deal with their feelings. Disruptions in peer relationships and academic learning are common. Pre-teens may feel powerless, frightened, and intensely angry with one or both parents. They are more likely than younger children to take active sides in ongoing battles between their parents. Adolescents tend to react either with depression, acting out, and emotional and social withdrawal from friends and school or with a developmental spurt, showing unexpected maturity, empathy, and compassion and providing significant help to one or both parents. School social adjustment and academic performance may be negatively affected.

The relative effects of different custody options are difficult to study, although in one 12-year follow-up study of low-income families with contested custody in divorce who had been randomly assigned to mediation or litigation, mediation resulted in greater continuing involvement with the nonresidential parent without an associated increase in coparenting conflict (Emery et al. 2001). Some research has found a positive correlation between joint legal custody and children's adjustment; however, parents' psychological well-being and the quality of the parent–child relationship are key variables. Divorcing parents who *request* joint custody are likely to be those who are more able to maintain a parental coalition and active involvement of both parents, despite the dissolution of the marriage. Fathers with joint custody are more likely to remain emotionally involved with and financially supportive of the children. If a judge awards joint custody against the wishes of one or both parents, severe conflict is likely to continue, to the detriment of the child. This is particularly true for infants and toddlers who are often forced into overnight visits at a time when separations may be traumatic. Single-parent custody relationships have been effective, particularly when contact with the noncustodial parent remains an option for the child. Even when the noncustodial parent has been unreliable or has acted violently, the child may continue to request visits. Unfortunately, divorce almost always has a detrimental effect on the relationship between the noncustodial parent and the child. Contacts become primarily social, and these parents rarely are partners in the child's discipline or education. There is evidence, however, for noncustodial fathers that the quality of paternal parenting and the child–father relationship are more important than frequency of contact (Amato and Gilbreth 1999).

Marital separation and divorce create social upheaval for the child. The standard of living typically declines, due to spreading the family income over two households instead of one, inadequate child support, and mothers who may be poorly equipped to enter the job market. When a stay-at-home mother must return to work, children may be traumatized by yet another separation. Reduced income may lead to a move to a more modest neighborhood, with resulting separation from familiar peers, neighbors, and school.

Divorce has phases that require repeated adjustment. Some children do poorly during the first year after divorce, a time that forces change on the parent as well as the child. Many parents, coping with their own anger, grief, depression, anxiety, and loneliness, as well as struggling with the financial settlement and the practicalities of maintaining separate households, are emotionally unavailable to their children and unable to provide consistent routine and discipline. Typically, hostility between parents decreases over time. Long-term child adjustment is dependent on the ability of the custodial parent to maintain a functional household, continue the child's relationship with the noncustodial parent, avoid severe economic hardship, and provide emotional nurturance to the child. Adolescents and young adults may experience delayed effects of divorce as they enter dating, falling in love, and marriage.

Although many boys are more oppositional, defiant, and aggressive following divorce than are girls, these behaviors typically predate the divorce. Preexisting symptoms may be exacerbated by parental separation, however. Boys suffer especially from loss of their father, who provides a male model and firmer discipline. Boys are more likely than girls to be exposed to parental fights, receive more inconsistent and negative discipline from divorced mothers, have mothers who report more stress and depression, and receive less positive support and nurturance from mothers, teachers, and peers after the divorce. Most children of divorced parents eventually must readjust to one or more new families, as one or both of their parents remarry. Remarriage of a custodial mother is associated with increased problems in the mother–daughter relationship but decreased behavioral symptoms in boys. Perhaps this is because stepfathers have stronger relationships with stepsons than with stepdaughters. Young adolescents who have functioned in parental roles often have special difficulty adjusting to a stepparent, who usurps some of their duties and privileges. Awareness of the parent's sexual activity is acutely embarrassing to teenagers.

Although some young adults who have faced divorce as children have significant consequences, the majority have resilient outcomes. Children of divorced families have been reported to have more subsequent behavioral problems, including substance use and difficulties with relationships, than those in intact families, although less so than previously believed. Age of the child, time since divorce, parenting styles, and degree of parental/family conflict likely influence these complex issues of postdivorce adjustment.

Interventions

Education regarding expectable reactions to divorce is useful for parents and children. A support group may reduce feelings of isolation and guilt, especially in communities where divorce is uncommon. Postdivorce groups or workshops based in schools offer services with less stigma. Parents Without Partners, a self-help group with chapters nationwide, offers companionship, advice, and moral support from adult peers, as well as educational programs and role models for children. Brief focused therapy can help children and parents deal with their feelings and aid parents in resolving conflict and establishing new lives. In a controlled trial with white, middle-class families undergoing divorce, a 6-year follow-up of a group and individual prevention program with mothers, with or without their school-age children, found that the adolescents from the intervention groups (compared with controls, who received reading material) had fewer mental disorders and fewer sexual partners. Among those initially at higher risk, the intervention subjects had fewer behavior problems and less substance use (Wolchik et al. 2002). Some states provide court-connected programs that offer or mandate evaluation, counseling, and crisis intervention and make recommendations to the judge regarding custody, visitation rights, and child support. Divorce and custody mediation is available as an effective alternative to the adversarial litigation process. However, in circumstances of abuse, violence, mental limitations or illness, the judicial system is appropriate for protection of children and parents. Children and parents with significant symptoms may require more extensive psychiatric evaluation including individual and/or family therapy. Parental psychiatric problems following divorce are associated with more difficulties for children; therefore, prompt treatment for these adults is critical.

Physical Illness in Parents or Siblings

When a family member is chronically or seriously ill, parental resources in time, money, and emotional energy available to other family members are reduced. In addition, nearly all children have at some time wished that something bad would happen to a parent or sibling. If that person then falls ill, the child may literally believe that he or she caused the illness. This "magical thinking" is normal in young children and appears under stress even at later developmental stages.

To the extent that an ill child receives special treatment, sibling rivalry is exacerbated. This may be overt or concealed by the child's guilt or parental shaming. A child or an adolescent often must take on extra chores to substitute for a parent or sibling. Parents can help by equalizing chores, discipline, privileges, and treats as much as developmental stages and physical condition permit.

Childhood disability and illness have an impact on the whole family system, although there is a paucity of systematic study. The sibling of a disabled child may be teased by peers. Correct information about the disability will facilitate coping. Some siblings of children with severe, chronic disabilities are more likely to have symptoms of aggression, depression, social isolation, and oppositional behavior. Families already stressed (e.g., by financial strain or single parenthood) are at higher risk for emotional or behavioral symptoms.

Death of a Family Member

The death of a family member, particularly a parent or primary caregiver, is a traumatic event for a child that can elicit strong emotional or behavioral responses. One in 20 children experiences the death of a parent. Bereaved children often experience depressed mood, sadness, longing for the deceased, appetite changes, irritability, social withdrawal, declining school performance, and sleep disturbances, although children's expressions of grief tend to be more intermittent than adults'. In the first 2 months after parental death, the effect can be profound and may lead to the development of major depression and suicidal ideation. However, the severity of these symptoms generally wanes over time. In a longitudinal study of the psychosocial functioning of bereaved children from stable families, the children appeared similar in function to healthy control subjects (Fristad et al. 1993). If the death occurred under traumatic circumstances, the expected anger and grief may escalate to *childhood traumatic grief,* including PTSD symptoms. If the death involves a child, the siblings must face their own grief in the context of their grieving parents' emotional withdrawal. Suicide-bereaved children have to address grief as well as the stigma and anguish surrounding suicide. Suicide-bereaved children experienced more anxiety, anger, and shame than children bereaved from parental death not caused by suicide (Cerel et al. 1999).

The terminal phase of the parental illness may, in fact, be more stressful for the child than the death. During this time, the child is exposed to the physical changes and painful consequences of life-threatening disease. The child also becomes aware of the irreversible nature of the illness and the likelihood of death. Parental illness changes the structure and organization of the family. Family roles and routines change, and family cohesiveness may suffer as the ill parent becomes less available physically and emotionally, and the other parent may be exhausted by caretaking and grief. Terminal phases of illness require more resources for care, which may jeopardize the family's financial stability. When a parent has been ill, the death may mark the end of a tragic and difficult period for the family and begin the process of healing and reorganization.

When a family member dies, the child should be allowed some choice in whether to attend the funeral (if developmentally appropriate). One study (Weller et al. 1988) showed that attendance at funeral activities did not result in increased psychiatric symptoms 2 months later. Extra support, such as an adult friend or relative, can be helpful through the funeral process, because the surviving parent is often too preoccupied with his or her own grief to be very available to the child. Children can mourn, although they may express their grief in behavior rather than verbally. If the child is especially vulnerable because of a psychiatric disorder or additional stressors, clinical judgment should influence the decision about how to handle the funeral, and extra therapeutic support may be needed.

Parents should explain death in a matter-of-fact, concrete way. Religious explanations should be used only if these are consistent with family beliefs. It is not wise to say that "death is like sleeping" or that "God took a person because He loved him (or her)" because children may then have fears of sleeping or of being taken by God. One could explain that body functions stop working when someone is very old or very sick. The magical thinking and egocentricity that are normal characteristics of children lead them to believe that they may be responsible for the death. They will often be too frightened or guilty to mention this and should be spontaneously reassured that they had nothing to do with the cause of the death.

The child's conceptualization of death plays a role in adjustment. As children mature, they gradually develop an understanding that death is universal and irreversible. Children younger than 2 or 3 years do not understand at all; they are simply made anxious by the separation. At ages 4–5 years, death seems reversible, like sleep or a long journey. Preschoolers believe that dead people can eat, sleep, and play, either in heaven or under the ground, and may view death as reversible, like sleep or a long trip. For 5- to 10-year-olds, death can be personified. A more realistic concept of death develops in children ages 10–11 years. Although by then most understand that death is universal, more than half of fourth graders do not yet clearly understand the irreversibility of death. Elementary school–age children tend to view death as a punishment for bad behavior. Although adolescents cognitively understand the meaning of death, they often do not accept their own mortality.

The longer-term effects of family bereavement depend on how well the surviving parents cope and are able to restore family life functioning. Open and honest expressiveness among mutually supportive family members facilitates this process. If the child's life is further disrupted by economic hardship or changes in school, home, and friends or the child's relationship with the deceased parent had been conflictual, the risk of significant adjustment problems may be increased.

Adoption

Adopted children are overrepresented in psychiatric treatment settings. Possible contributing factors to the higher rate of psychiatric referral of adopted children include genetic or prenatal risks from the birth parents; disruptions, trauma, or neglect in the child's early life; adoptive home problems (such as unrealistic expectations by both the adoptive parents and the child, the parents' negative feelings about the inability to conceive, parental and grandparental favoritism toward natural children, criticism from the extended family, poor communication); and the child's unresolved feelings about being given up for adoption or identity issues. The understanding of temperament (see Chapter 2) emphasizes the importance of "goodness of fit" between parent and child. To the extent that there is a genetic contribution to temperament, adopted children may be more likely to be mismatched with one or both parents, increasing the risk of behavior and emotional problems.

Children adopted past infancy are at higher risk for psychiatric problems as a result of the experiences that led to placement for adoption. These children have endured not only the loss of their parent(s) or primary attachment figure, but perhaps also neglect, abuse, and frequent changes of caregiver. Some children adopted after spending their first years in a residential nursery or orphanage are capable of forming stable affectionate relationships with their adoptive parents, but many show significant social and attentional problems and attachment difficulties.

It is normal for children and adolescents, even those who have not been adopted, to go through stages of questioning whether they are with their "real" parents and whether another set of parents would be better. It is important for adoptive parents not to take these stages too seriously or personally. Although there is not a clear consensus of when the best time is to disclose adoption status, the child's cognitive functioning should be taken into account. The trend is increasingly toward "open" adoption, where children are told early and there may be contact with the birth mother.

■ ADOLESCENT PREGNANCY

Demographics

In 2006 data reported by the Guttmacher Institute (www.guttmacher.org), the rate of pregnancy among U.S. girls ages 15–19 years was 7%. This rate was up slightly from 2005, the year of lowest rate in U.S. teens in 30 years. The teenage birthrate was 42 births per 1,000 in 2006. The proportion of teen pregnancies ending in abortion continued to decline, to 32% of pregnancies. There are large disparities by state of residence and by race, with adolescent girls of color at higher risk for unintended pregnancy.

The Mother

Adolescents who become pregnant are not a uniform group; they differ by race, socioeconomic status, and age. In studies controlled for academic aptitude and financial status, teenage mothers are less likely to complete high school, less likely to achieve a stable and well-paying job, more likely to be dependent on public assistance, and less likely to enter a stable marriage than their peers. In addition, teenage mothers are more likely to have anemia and hypertension. Interestingly, those who are able to finish high school, avoid another pregnancy in their teens, and marry do not show negative effects at long-term follow-up when compared with peers who delayed their first pregnancy.

The Child

Lack of adequate prenatal care is a risk factor for prematurity, low birth weight, and neonatal mortality, especially for mothers younger than age 15 years. Children of teenage mothers have higher postneonatal mortality rates and more subsequent illnesses and injuries.

Children, especially sons, of teenage parents appear to be at a developmental disadvantage and may be at higher risk for emotional problems, hyperactivity, aggression, school failure, and incarceration. The daughters of adolescent mothers are more likely to become pregnant before age 18 years than offspring of mothers in their 20s. Relative contributions of poor prenatal care, genetic factors, parental limited education, and suboptimal parenting because of immaturity, financial stresses, and living in disadvantaged neighborhoods with low-quality schools are difficult to tease out.

Interventions

Once an adolescent becomes pregnant, nonjudgmental support for the young woman and her family, along with practical and educational assistance, may facilitate making an informed decision among adoption, abortion, and raising the child. Young mothers are most satisfied with the outcome of their pregnancy when they receive parental support for their decision. Adolescents may not be able to anticipate or understand the consequences of the pregnancy and so require continued support. For teenage mothers raising a child, outreach programs offering prenatal care, child care, parenting training, assistance in completing high school, further academic or vocational training, and enrichment programs such as Head Start for the children can positively affect long-term outcome.

Even a negative pregnancy test provides an opportunity for medical and psychosocial intervention, because these adolescents are likely to become pregnant and are more likely than their peers to have multiple partners. Screening for sexually transmitted diseases, provision of effective contraception, and education regarding "safe sex" and the psychosocial impact of pregnancy should follow a pregnancy test (or completed pregnancy) in all adolescents, whether positive or negative.

■ OBESITY

Clinical Description

Obesity, or medically significant overweight, caused by excess body fat, is coded on DSM-IV-TR Axis III. Body mass index (BMI; weight in kg/height in m²), the most appropriate measure to screen for childhood obesity, has norms by age and gender. A BMI greater than the 95th percentile is defined as obesity.

Epidemiology

The prevalence of childhood obesity is increasing dramatically, and has been called an epidemic. Data from the 2007–2008 National Health and Nutrition Examination Survey found an estimated 17% of youth to be obese. African American youth and Hispanic boys are at greatest risk for both obesity and overweight (BMI greater than 85th percentile).

Etiology

Genetic, medical, and family environmental factors contribute to the development of obesity. Parental obesity greatly increases the risk. Girls are more likely to become obese during adolescence because body fat typically increases, in contrast to males, who tend to lose body fat as adolescents. There is little evidence that metabolic rates differ significantly between obese children and those of normal weight. Genetic factors may influence weight gain, but do not explain the dramatic increase in childhood obesity over the past 30 years. During this period, physical activity decreased while intake of fat and refined sugar rose.

Course and Prognosis

Obesity in middle childhood (especially if it persists through adolescence) predicts adult obesity. Childhood obesity can result in medical complications, including cardiovascular disease and diabetes. Severe liver disease with hepatitis and fibrosis may result. Obstructive sleep apnea as a consequence of weight gain can lead to nighttime hypoxemia, cardiac arrhythmias, and right heart failure. Obesity carries a social stigma as well. Children have more difficulty making and keeping friends, negatively affecting levels of self-esteem.

Evaluation and Differential Diagnosis

A pediatric examination is indicated to rule out rare specific chromosomal (e.g., Klinefelter's syndrome, Prader-Willi syndrome) or endocrine (e.g., hypothyroidism, Cushing's disease) causes of obesity. The clinician must also understand the eating habits and activity level of the entire family and determine how each caregiver perceives the problem. There should be unanimity among family members because the patient will otherwise receive mixed messages that will undermine treatment. Many parents (often themselves overweight) do not perceive their children as having weight problems.

Treatment

Multimodal treatment of obesity combines cognitive-behavioral modification in a group setting, balanced diet, and exercise, in collaboration with the pediatrician. Traditional psychotherapy is not effective in the treatment of obesity per se. Some families need multimodal psychological and practical supports. Contingency management is useful in the treatment of obesity in younger children: a chart is used to record points earned for self-monitoring, control of eating, and exercise that may be exchanged for rewards or negotiated backup reinforcers. Adolescents are taught to keep a detailed diary, including food intake and events and feelings preceding eating. They learn self-reinforcement (making positive statements about themselves when they resist temptation) and coping strategies. "Cognitive restructuring" eliminates negative and self-defeating statements about eating and weight. An unmotivated youngster can easily cheat. The most difficult problem is long-term maintenance of appropriate weight. Cognitive-behavioral modification includes "relapse prevention" techniques to learn to identify high-risk situations, use coping strategies such as problem solving and assertiveness, and avoid turning a small slip into a catastrophic lapse.

Nutritional education is essential for both parents and children. The "Traffic Light Diet" (Epstein and Wing 1987) identifies foods as green (to be consumed freely), yellow (to be eaten with caution), and red (to be avoided entirely). A weight-reduction diet must be nutritionally adequate. Extreme diets may have more serious consequences in developing children than in adults.

Family involvement in the treatment of obesity is essential, because parents control access to food, at least in younger children, and dispense most rewards and punishments. If both parent and child are obese, treatment of the child's obesity is more likely to succeed if the parent is treated simultaneously *and* loses weight. Interestingly, the child's maintenance of weight loss does not seem to depend on the parent's maintenance. Modeling is apparently important in initial weight loss, but contingent reinforcement and child self-regulation are important in maintenance. For adolescents, separate treatment of the parent may be more effective.

Exercise increases calorie expenditure, increases basal metabolism rate (thus avoiding the decrease that otherwise accompanies calorie restriction), suppresses appetite, and reduces the medical complications of obesity. Sensible diet plus incorporating increased physical activity into everyday routines, or "lifestyle exercise," are more effective in maintaining weight loss than more intensive aerobic exercise programs, which have lower long-term adherence.

■ PHYSICALLY ILL CHILDREN AND ADOLESCENTS

Developmental Factors in Reaction to Acute Illness, Hospitalization, and Surgery

The emotional response to illness is dependent on the child's stage of development, the amount of discomfort, the type of treatment and its side effects, the practical limitations that result from the illness, premorbid psychiatric problems in the patient, and the child's level of understanding. Parents affect the child's reaction through their own coping mechanisms and the support they provide. Physicians can usually predict the most stressful times in the course of an illness and should take these opportunities to provide additional emotional support. Innovations such as parental rooming-in, unlimited parental visiting, permitting parents to be present while the child is sedated preoperatively, and outpatient surgery to avoid hospital admissions have reduced emotional aftereffects. The use of primary nurses and child development specialists in the hospital has also facilitated children's adjustment. Preparation, individualized to coping style and developmental level, may be done via talks explaining procedures, visits, books, puppet shows, and films.

Infancy

Hospitalized infants younger than 6 months are most upset by the change in the usual routine. It is helpful to have the parents do as much of the caregiving as possible and to arrange for consistent nurses. For the older infant who has formed strong differential attachments, separation is traumatic, and stranger anxiety adds to the infant's distress. Infants respond to the emotional reactions of the primary caregivers. An anxious, tense mother will be less able to soothe and comfort her child than one who is calmer and in better control. The infant's immature cognitive development exacerbates the problem because explanations are of no use. Infants do not recognize that they have an illness or disability and simply respond to discomfort by crying or becoming irritable. Fortunately, most pediatric hospital settings encourage parents to "live in" while their infant is hospitalized. In the absence of an attachment figure, the baby's physical agitation, refusal to eat, and inability to sleep may have serious medical consequences.

Early Childhood

Hospitalized children ages 1–3 years may react to separation from their parents by rejecting parents when they visit, being aggressive toward medical staff, regressing in bowel and bladder control, and/or refusing to eat. If parents are absent, children may develop depression, sleep disturbance, diarrhea, or vomiting. Maximizing parental presence and providing the child with familiar items from home, especially the child's favorite toy or blanket (transitional object), are helpful. Developmentally, this is a time of increasing exploration and autonomy. Unfortunately, toddlers frequently attempt to master their environment by becoming more oppositional. Offering the child as much predictability, consistency, and control (choices) as possible can reduce distress and resistance.

For children ages 3–5 years, separation from parents by hospitalization is difficult, even for a child who is comfortably able to separate in other circumstances. Anesthesia and surgery are especially frightening because of normal developmental fears of bodily injury. Children believe that illness and painful treatments are punishment for real or fantasized misbehavior. When possible, preparation by simple explanations and a visit to the hospital may help. Frequent presence of a parent is important. When understandably anxious parents attempt to protect the child's health by limiting the child's activities, including delaying school enrollment, an unintended consequence may be to increase passivity, dependence, and fearfulness in the child.

School Age

Children ages 6–12 years usually tolerate acute illness and hospitalization relatively well, especially when they are prepared, their parents are present, and the child's preceding development was on course. They may still have irrational explanations of illness (e.g., that they are being punished or that their parents were unable to protect them). Peer relationships become paramount during this period, and comparisons of physical appearance and capabilities are likely. Medically ill children become aware of their differences and limitations; occasionally their friendships are affected. School attendance and participation are major developmental tasks of childhood; medically ill children have more academic problems than their non–medically ill peers. These problems may be caused by the effects of the illness and its treatment, decreased expectations in the classroom, school absences, or psychosocial stressors. Reactions often include regression or oppositional behavior.

Adolescence

Adolescents have more realistic fears regarding the outcome of illness, such as changes in appearance or inability to continue favorite activities. An injury may make impossible a planned career (e.g., sports, the military). Loss of autonomy and privacy is especially painful for adolescents. The adolescent should be given some control over treatment to avoid struggles between the patient and the caregiver and to convey that the adolescent's opinions are important. Occasionally, noncompliance can be an expression of suicidal ideation, particularly when the consequences are life threatening. Physical appearance and sexuality emerge as priorities during adolescence, and patients with sequelae of illness, injury, or treatment need additional support.

Chronic Illness

The Child's Reaction

Chronic illness can lead to interference with academic, social, and recreational development. Autonomy and control of the child's own body are jeopardized, and self-esteem may be lowered. Especially in adolescence, peers have little tolerance for differences in appearance or behavior. Children and adolescents with chronic illness without disability are twice as likely as control children to have a psychiatric disorder. Those with disability as well as chronic illness are even more likely to have emotional and attention-deficit disorders, social isolation, and school performance problems. The nature of the disability does not appear to be significant unless it involves the central nervous system. Central nervous system disorders are even more likely to have psychiatric sequelae. Episodic illness is more stressful than persistent medical disorders because of the unpredictability of the problem and the need to respond to sudden changes in physical condition. Psychiatric distress may present as an increase in dependent, fearful behavior; an escalation in risk-taking or acting-out behaviors; or, in older children and adolescents, a tendency to become angry, hostile, and isolative. Somatoform disorders are another manifestation of psychiatric illness. Headaches, recurrent abdominal pain, limb pain, chest pain, or fatigue that are affected by psychological factors interact with symptoms of medical disorders and may be difficult to distinguish. The combination can lead to increased physical disability. Catastrophic injury and devastating illness can lead to symptoms of PTSD in both the pediatric patient and the parent. Support should be provided to the child, parent, and medical staff. Psychiatric disorder is not inevitable in chronically ill children and adolescents. Fewer than one-third of those with chronic illness have mental health problems or difficulties with social or school adjustment (Cadman et al. 1987).

The Parents' Reaction

The most critical factor in the child's ability to cope with chronic illness is the response of the family. Medical illness in a child tends to exaggerate all the strengths and weaknesses of the family. At the time of diagnosis, the parents must go through a period of mourning with stages similar to those following a death: anger, denial, grief, and resignation. Medical problems in a child may be viewed by the parent (and others) as a negative reflection on the parent. Parents feel guilty, especially for genetic diseases or pregnancy complications. The psychological status of parents is strongly related to their perception of the child's illness. Clinicians must, therefore, attend to the parent's understanding of the disorder and all of its implications. Realistic additional caregiving and financial burdens may stress parents beyond their ability to cope. Chronic illness increases the strain on a marriage. The parents' anger, resentment, guilt, and/or denial may interfere with their ability to communicate with each other and to work with the pediatric team. Parents may distance themselves from the child, become overly close or intrusive, or alternate between the two. Mothers of children with chronic illness are at increased risk for depression.

The Terminally Ill Child or Adolescent

When a young person is dying, parents or medical personnel may make misguided attempts to "protect" the child. These are perceived as in the best interests of the child but more often relate to the difficulties adults have with a child's death. Although young patients may not fully understand their clinical situation, children are astute observers of emotions in their parents, nurses, and doctors. If the child is not dealt with honestly, his or her imagination can be even worse than the reality. Children understand the permanence of death by age 10 or 11 years, although they may not understand the relationship between it and the biological aspects of their illness. Parents or physicians may need to tell children about their terminal illness in stages, as understanding progresses and the child is able to cope with the knowledge. Children are often more concerned about immediate details of treatment and its effect on them than about ultimate survival. The child or adolescent should be given the opportunity, but not be forced, to talk about disease, disability, or death. Drawing, painting, or doll play may be useful symbolic outlets and means of communication.

The terminal phase of an illness leads to a recapitulation in parents of the feelings of denial, anger, grief, depression, and guilt that followed the initial diagnosis. Discussions about death between parent and child should be encouraged as a way to prepare the child, answer his or her questions and fears, and say good-bye. If a child is terminally ill for a long time, anticipatory mourning may be completed, and some parents gradually detach, leaving the child no emotional place in the family. Similarly, physicians may inadvertently avoid the child and family when aggressive treatment is no longer an option and the medical team is resigned to the patient's death. Alternatively, if a child who is expected to die recovers, parents often experience a "Damocles syndrome," living in constant fear of disease exacerbation and death. Other parents come into conflict with medical caregivers by demanding additional active treatments that are medically considered to be futile. A hospital ethics committee or palliative care consultation may be helpful.

The Child or Adolescent With AIDS

Children infected with human immunodeficiency virus (HIV) have even more difficulties than the typical chronically ill child. Even now, these young people may be stigmatized by peers, teachers, other adults in the community, potential foster parents, and even health care personnel. Poverty is common, and parenting may be poor. The psychiatric effects of the disease itself are often added to associated factors that put the child at risk, including an HIV-infected mother who may be dying or dead or adolescent behavior problems that led to unprotected intercourse and/or injection drug use. The sequelae of central nervous system infection by the virus (delayed development, cognitive impairment, and organic mood and behavior disorders) add to the burden of illness. Counseling HIV-positive adolescents regarding sexual behavior and their plans for the future is essential.

Adherence to Treatment

Lack of adherence to or compliance with medical procedures and regimens can be a major problem in the care of children and adolescents. Factors in the child and parent, family dynamics, the nature of the treatment, and the relationship between the child and family and the medical team can all contribute to poor adherence. Severe noncompliance may warrant a full psychiatric evaluation and treatment of individual psychiatric disorders and/or family dysfunction.

Adherence is facilitated by giving the child or adolescent as much responsibility for the treatment as possible, gradually increasing responsibility as interest, understanding, and behavior control improve. The child should participate in decision making and be offered as many choices as possible. Explanations can be targeted to the child's ability to understand. The normal compulsiveness of children ages 6–12 years can be harnessed to develop a habit of charting or record keeping related to the treatment. If children or adolescents are able to develop their own relationships with medical personnel, compliance may be facilitated by avoiding the struggles for independence inherent in the parent–child relationship. Adults should minimize power struggles and, whenever possible, negotiate and solve problems with the young person. At times, a child's noncompliance signals a parent's ambivalence or even opposition to treatment.

Treatment

Psychotherapy

Supportive individual, family, and/or group education and psychotherapy are often valuable for the patient and parents. Instruction in social problem-solving and coping skills may be beneficial.

Support Groups

Support groups for children and adolescents and for parents, both separately and as families, may be helpful. These groups provide emotional support and inform the patient and the family about challenges the disease is likely to present. Chronically ill children may benefit from disease-specific camps and recreation programs with medical supervision, which permit them more normal activities and provide a respite for parents.

Pharmacotherapy

Indications for the use of pharmacotherapy in medically ill children and adolescents do not differ from those in routine psychiatric cases. Drug choice and management decisions are, however, affected by the illness and should be made in conjunction with the pediatric specialist. Risk of side effects is higher because of both medication interactions and illness. Disorders that are the direct consequence of medical illness, including delirium and organic affective states, should be addressed by treating the primary cause. Situational and anticipatory anxiety related to medical procedures may benefit from hydroxyzine, diazepam, or alprazolam if psychosocial intervention is insufficient. Treatable depression should be actively sought, because depression is not an inevitable response to illness and may dramatically impede recovery.

Behavior Modification

Techniques such as behavior contracting with contingency management and self-monitoring with self-reinforcement are invaluable in improving medical and behavioral compliance. Children who refuse or are unable to swallow oral medication can be taught to take pills using instruction, modeling, contingent rewards, and a behavior-shaping protocol that involves successively larger candies or placebos (Pelco et al. 1987).

Cognitive-behavioral techniques can be used to ameliorate a variety of chronic physical symptoms and symptom-related behaviors. For example, in treating headache, the antecedents and consequences of pain are determined (by keeping a pain diary, if the child is old enough), and attempts are made to modify events and situations that precipitate or positively reinforce pain. The clinician works with the patient, parents, teachers, pediatrician, and significant others to emphasize functioning normally despite pain as well as stress management techniques. Reductions in pain and pain-related behaviors give patients a sense of control and mastery and a return to age-appropriate activities. *Stress inoculation* helps to prevent anxiety in children before medical and dental procedures and reduces anxiety, pain, or discomfort connected to repeated procedures such as chemotherapy injections, bone marrow aspirations, and spinal taps in chronically ill children. Stress inoculation consists of multicomponent cognitive-behavioral approaches, including education, modeling procedures, systematic desensitization, hypnosis, contingency management, imagery, and breathing exercises.

Hypnosis is readily used in children, who are generally more hypnotizable than adults. Different techniques are appropriate for children of different ages. Hypnosis is used in treating physical symptoms with a psychological component or managing severe physical symptoms (pain, nausea) associated with a medical disorder or treatment.

Relaxation training for children and adolescents is used to manage pain in pediatric migraine, juvenile rheumatoid arthritis, and hemophilia. These techniques can result in decreased subjective experience of pain, reduced need for analgesics, and even improved mood, self-esteem, and physical and social functioning. Relaxation techniques are also used in treating asthma or cystic fibrosis in patients who hyperventilate.

■ CHILDREN OF PSYCHIATRICALLY ILL PARENTS

Risks and Resilience

Children of mentally ill parents are at increased risk for psychiatric disturbance, due to both genetic factors and the effect of mental illness on parenting skills and family environment. Child outcome may be affected by parental marital discord with conflict over child rearing and an inability to provide adequate support in the face of life challenges. Parents may be less affectionate, particularly when struggling with depression, leading to impairment that can extend across generations. Poor decision making may result in inadequate supervision and exposure to danger. Occasionally the parent's psychiatric illness involves the child (e.g., a delusion about the child). Family disruption may lead to divorce or placement of the child outside of the home. The risk of psychopathology in the child is related to the severity and chronicity of psychiatric illness in the parent. Both assortative mating and a contagion effect may result in two parents with a mental disorder, increasing the likelihood that their offspring will suffer a psychiatric illness.

Children are particularly distressed when their parents are admitted to a psychiatric hospital. Younger children may show sleep disturbance, decreased appetite, attention-seeking behavior, separation anxiety, crying (especially at bedtime), and social withdrawal. Adolescents are more able to verbalize their fears, guilt, and concerns about themselves and their parents.

Children whose parents have a mood disorder have an increased (but by no means inevitable) incidence of depressive symptoms and nonspecific behavior and emotional disturbance. These children are more likely to experience a variety of internalizing symptoms including recurrent feelings of guilt, interpersonal problems, and difficulties with attachment. Children of schizophrenic parents are more likely to have abnormalities in attention and information processing, even before overt symptoms emerge. Children of patients with anxiety disorders have a markedly increased risk for an anxiety disorder themselves, as well as for symptoms such as fears and worries, school difficulties, somatic complaints, and social isolation.

A significant minority of children of alcoholic parents have increased behavior problems, especially conduct problems, hyperactivity, impulsivity, hypersensitivity to stimuli, poor self-control, inattention, and emotional symptoms such as anxiety and depression. Prenatal alcohol exposure is a common nongenetic cause of mental retardation and can contribute to the development of learning and language disabilities. Children of alcohol abusers are more likely to develop alcohol problems themselves, and the disinhibition associated with substance use places them at greater risk for suicide, accidents, unplanned pregnancy, HIV exposure, and school failure.

Some "resilient" children not only resist and cope with unusual stress but also thrive and succeed despite adversity. Protective factors include a cohesive and emotionally supportive family environment and external support systems, such as caring extended family members, other adults, and/or institutional supports (e.g., school or community agencies). These children have a strong commitment to extracurricular activities and interpersonal relationships and tend to be confident and self-reliant. They are realistic in their assessment of the family and its limitations, and understand their own coping style when dealing with parental psychiatric illness.

Adolescence is a particularly high-risk period for the development of major depression in the offspring of parents with mood disorder. Successful adaptation is characterized by close, confiding relationships; persistence and success in school and work; and involvement in activities. They are able to separate themselves, cognitively and emotionally, from their parent and their parent's illness, while often functioning as caregivers in the family. Coping skills include accurate cognitive appraisal of the stress to be dealt with, realistic assessment of their responsibilities and powers, and an understanding of the parent's illness (especially that they are not responsible for their parent's depression). Remission in maternal depression with treatment is associated with a decrease in symptoms in the child (Weissman et al. 2006).

Interventions

Parents can promote resilient traits in their children and moderate the emotional consequences of their psychiatric illness. Communication between spouses and among family members improves the level of understanding and reduces guilt and emotional upset. Children should be referred to appropriate support groups. Individual strengths in the child should be encouraged and nurtured. When parents are receiving psychiatric treatment, the treating clinician should be alert to possible effects of the illness on the children. Parental psychiatric hospitalization is particularly stressful. There should be at least one family session near the time of admission to explain the need for hospitalization and the anticipated treatment course. Optimally, a member of the treatment team interviews each child to assess developmental level, school performance, peer relationships, coping skills for dealing with and understanding parental illness, and the possible presence of psychiatric symptoms. Efforts can be made to enrich and strengthen the child's support system. Placement with a relative or in foster care may be necessary until the parent can resume child-care responsibilities.

■ REFERENCES

Amato PR, Gilbreth JG: Nonresident fathers and children's well-being: a meta-analysis. J Marriage Fam 61:557–573, 1999

American Psychiatric Association: Diagnostic and Statistical Manual of Mental Disorders, 4th Edition, Text Revision. Washington, DC, American Psychiatric Association, 2000

Buehler C, Krishnakumar A, Stone G, et al: Interparental conflict styles and youth problem behaviors: a two-sample replication study. J Marriage Fam 60:119–132, 1998

Cadman D, Boyle M, Szatmari P, et al: Chronic illness, disability, and mental and social well-being: findings of the Ontario Child Health Study. Pediatrics 79:805–813, 1987

Cerel J, Fristad MA, Weller EB, et al: Suicide-bereaved children and adolescents: a controlled longitudinal examination. J Am Acad Child Adolesc Psychiatry 38:672–679, 1999

Cohen JA, Deblinger E, Mannarino AP, et al: A multisite, randomized controlled trial for children with sexual abuse-related PTSD symptoms. J Am Acad Child Adolesc Psychiatry 43:393–402, 2004

Emery RE, Laumann-Billings L, Waldron MC, et al: Child custody mediation and litigation: custody, contact, and coparenting 12 years after initial dispute resolution. J Consult Clin Psychol 69:323–332, 2001

Epstein LH, Wing RR: Behavioral treatment of childhood obesity. Psychol Bull 101:331–342, 1987

Fristad MA, Jedel R, Weller RA, et al: Psychosocial functioning in children after the death of a parent. Am J Psychiatry 150:511–513, 1993

Miller AL, Rathus JH, Linehan MM: Dialectical Behavior Therapy With Suicidal Adolescents. New York, Guilford, 2007

Pelco LE, Kissel RC, Parrish JM, et al: Behavioral management of oral medication administration difficulties among children: a review of literature with case illustrations. J Dev Behav Pediatr 8:90–96, 1987

Weissman MM, Pilowsky DJ, Wickramartne PJ, et al: Remissions in maternal depression and child psychopathology: a STAR*D-child report. JAMA 295:1389–1398, 2006

Weller EB, Weller RA, Fristad MA, et al: Should children attend their parent's funeral? J Am Acad Child Adolesc Psychiatry 27:559–562, 1988

Wolchik SA, Sandler IN, Millsap RE, et al: Six-year follow-up of preventive interventions for children of divorce: a randomized controlled trial. JAMA 288:1874–1881, 2002

■ ADDITIONAL READING

American Academy of Child and Adolescent Psychiatry: Practice parameter for the psychiatric assessment and management of physically ill children and adolescents. J Am Acad Child Adolesc Psychiatry 48:213–233, 2009

American Academy of Child and Adolescent Psychiatry: Practice parameter for the assessment and treatment of children and adolescents with posttraumatic stress disorder. J Am Acad Child Adolesc Psychiatry 49:413–430, 2010

American Academy of Child and Adolescent Psychiatry: Practice parameter for the psychiatric assessment and treatment of children and adolescents with suicidal behavior. J Am Acad Child Adolesc Psychiatry 40 (7 suppl): 24S–51S, 2001

Beardslee WR, Martin JL: Children of parents with psychiatric and substance abuse disorders, in Dulcan's Textbook of Child and Adolescent Psychiatry. Edited by Dulcan MK. Washington, DC, American Psychiatric Publishing, 2010, pp 623–635

Cohen JA, Mannarino AP: Bereavement and Traumatic Grief, in Dulcan's Textbook of Child and Adolescent Psychiatry. Edited by Dulcan MK. Washington, DC, American Psychiatric Publishing, 2010, pp 509–516

Goldstein TR, Brent DA: Youth suicide, in Dulcan's Textbook of Child and Adolescent Psychiatry. Edited by Dulcan MK. Washington, DC, American Psychiatric Publishing, 2010, pp 531–542

Joshi PT, Daniolos PT, Salpekar JA: Child abuse and neglect, in Dulcan's Textbook of Child and Adolescent Psychiatry. Edited by Dulcan MK. Washington, DC, American Psychiatric Publishing, 2010, pp 479–494

Kelly JB: Children's adjustment in conflicted marriage and divorce: a decade review of research. J Am Acad Child Adolesc Psychiatry 39:963–973, 2000

Martini DR: Psychiatric emergencies, in Dulcan's Textbook of Child and Adolescent Psychiatry. Edited by Dulcan MK. Washington, DC, American Psychiatric Publishing, 2010, pp 583–594

Walsh F: Family transitions: challenges and resilience, in Dulcan's Textbook of Child and Adolescent Psychiatry. Edited by Dulcan MK. Washington, DC, American Psychiatric Publishing, 2010, pp 595–606

8

PSYCHOPHARMACOLOGY

■ SPECIAL ISSUES FOR CHILDREN AND ADOLESCENTS

General Principles

In the treatment of psychiatric disturbances in children and adolescents, psychopharmacology may be a key part of a multimodal treatment plan, the primary intervention, or an adjunct to other forms of treatment. The clinician must educate the family regarding the disorder, treatment options, and the child's needs at each developmental stage. The clinician also must consider the meaning of the prescription and administration of a drug to the child, family, and the child's teachers and peer group.

The clinical practice of pediatric psychopharmacology is impeded by the relative lack of double-blind randomized placebo-controlled trials. Many medications that appeared to be effective in anecdotal reports, case series, and open trials were not shown to be more effective than placebo in double-blind studies. In evaluating the medical literature on drug effects, it is important to distinguish between *statistically* significant and *clinically* significant effects: to know whether the target symptoms are reduced to near-normal levels or merely changed and to determine the clinical meaning of the change. Because groups are heterogeneous, some patients' conditions may improve and others may worsen, resulting in nonsignificant group data. Alternatively, statistically significant group changes may translate into only modest improvement in individual patient functioning and may not be worth the effort, expense, and potential risk of the treatment.

Simultaneous use of more than one medication ("polypharmacy") should be cautious and judicious, due to the increased risk of significant side effects, toxic drug interactions, and difficulty assessing effectiveness.

Developmental Toxicity

The interactions between drug treatment and physical, cognitive, social, and emotional development may produce unique or especially severe side effects. All psychotropic medications have the potential for cognitive toxicity. Because some drug treatments last for years, there is a risk of chronic and cumulative effects. Cognitive blunting can impair developing academic skills, social skills, and self-esteem even before physical side effects are observed, especially in young children. Young patients may have behavioral toxicity (i.e., the worsening of preexisting behaviors or affective states or the development of new symptoms). Behavioral toxicity typically abates after dose adjustments or change of drug.

Indications and Dosage

Once a drug is approved for any indication, the U.S. Food and Drug Administration (FDA) regulates only the company's advertising of the drug, not the prescribing behavior of physicians. Because in the past, pharmaceutical companies had little incentive to test drugs in children, the majority of psychopharmacological agents and indications (and most drugs used in pediatrics as well) lack pediatric labeling and are "unapproved" or "off-label" for children. As a result, the FDA guidelines as published in the *Physicians' Desk Reference* (PDR) cannot be relied on for appropriate indications, age ranges, or doses for children. Although lack of approval for an age group or a disorder does not imply improper or illegal use, it is prudent to inform the family of these labeling issues, as well as of evidence in the literature for safe and effective use. The physician should make clinical judgments based on the medical literature rather than the PDR.

Dosage may be determined by titration using effectiveness and side effects, within guidelines based on age, weight, or blood levels, or by extrapolation from adult doses. Although it is ideal for pediatric drug doses to be derived from data on children, these dosage studies are rare. A useful general principle for dosing is "start low and go slow."

The age-dependent processes of drug absorption, distribution, protein binding, metabolism, and elimination influence optimal dose size and schedule. Young children absorb some drugs more rapidly than do adults, leading to higher peak levels. Age-related factors that may influence distribution include uptake by actively growing tissue and proportional size of organs and tissue masses. Prior to puberty, children have, compared with adults, relatively more body water and less fat (which serves as a reservoir for lipid-soluble compounds) (Vitiello 2008). In children, drugs such as lithium (which are primarily distributed in body water) have a proportionally larger volume of distribution and therefore a lower concentration. By age 1 year, glomerular filtration rate and renal tubular secretion mechanisms reach adult levels. Hepatic enzyme activity develops early, and the rate of drug metabolism is then related to liver size. Both kidney and liver parenchyma in children are larger than in adults, relative to body size (Vitiello 2008). Therefore, compared with adults or older adolescents, children generally require a larger dose per kilogram of body weight of drugs that are primarily metabolized by the liver. They may also require divided doses to minimize fluctuations in blood level. Compared with adults, children also tend to have less protein binding of drugs, leaving a greater proportion of the drug biologically active.

Outcome

Assessing the risk-benefit ratio, especially for long-term treatment, is particularly complicated in children and adolescents. Many scientific unknowns persist regarding drug effects during development. Evaluation is complicated by a variety of nonpharmacological effects, including nonspecific therapeutic effects of evaluation and treatment, expectancy in the patient, parent, or teacher, changes in the environment, and the natural course of the disorder (e.g., the waxing and waning of symptoms in Tourette's disorder).

The clinician must specify target symptoms and obtain emotional, behavioral, and physical baseline and posttreatment data. Treatment effects can be assessed by interviews of and rating scales by the patient, the parent, and other caregivers (e.g., teachers, inpatient nurses); direct observation in the office, waiting room, or classroom; physical examination; and, as appropriate, specific cognitive, learning, or laboratory tests. The clinician must actively seek both therapeutic and adverse effects because many young patients will not report them spontaneously, and parents may not notice.

The interactions between treatment and the environment raise complex issues for children and adolescents. To assess medication effects in a child or adolescent, the clinician must evaluate and monitor the adult and peer environments as well as the patient. It is important to know what a clinical change and the therapeutic contacts mean to the patient and to family members.

The adults (parents, teachers, or staff in an inpatient unit or residential treatment setting) who care for children may misinterpret the youngster's response to the environment as indicating a need for medication or an improvement that is a result of medication. Some of these adults mistakenly seek to use psychotropic medication alone to control or eliminate a child's troublesome behavior, instead of investigating the family or institutional dynamics that may be provoking and maintaining such behavior or implementing more time-consuming, difficult, and expensive therapeutic or behavioral management strategies or changes in living situation.

It is important to give a medication an adequate trial for long enough (varies with each drug) and at a sufficient dose to determine effectiveness before switching to or adding another drug.

Adherence to Treatment

Effective treatment requires a therapeutic alliance and the cooperation of the patient, parents, school personnel, and often other caregivers. Compliance with a treatment regimen can be reduced by factors such as lack of perceived need for treatment, failure to understand the disorder, carelessness, lack of money, misunderstanding of instructions, or refusal to cooperate. Overly complex schedules of drug administration may make accurate administration nearly impossible. Media attention to alleged inappropriate use of medications has made some families and teachers highly resistant to pharmacotherapy.

Some children cannot or will not swallow pills. Some drugs are available in elixir or dissolving tablet form or can be dissolved in juice or sprinkled on pudding or applesauce. Problems with this method of administration may include unpleasant taste, chemical interaction resulting in precipitation of the medication, and inaccurate dosing. A behavior modification program to shape pill-swallowing behavior is available on the web at http://www.aboutourkids.org/articles/pill_swallowing_made_easy.

Ethical Issues

The careful clinician attempts to balance the risks of medication, the risks of the untreated disorder, and the expected benefits of medication relative to other treatments. With the exception of drugs used for ADHD, it is generally preferable to accumulate substantial clinical experience with a new drug in adults before it is used with children and young adolescents.

Consent for pharmacotherapy in children is a complex issue that can be made even more difficult if the parents or guardians are in conflict (e.g., in angry divorces or with children in the custody of child welfare). Informed consent is best considered an ongoing process rather than a single event. "Assent" to medication use is considered possible to obtain from a patient older than 7 years with more complex understanding at older ages. Formal consent forms are less useful than a documented discussion of therapeutic options with potential risks and benefits and an opportunity for questions and answers. Published information sheets for parents, youth, and teachers are available to supplement discussions with the physician about specific medications (Dulcan 2007).

■ STIMULANTS

The number of available stimulant preparations (Table 8–1) has increased dramatically. They include a variety of forms of methylphenidate and amphetamine.

Indications and Efficacy

Stimulant medications, including various formulations of methylphenidate, dexmethylphenidate, dextroamphetamine, amphetamine mixed salts, and lisdexamfetamine (see Table 8–1), are the first-line treatment for *ADHD*. The primary indication for stimulants is in the treatment of symptoms of ADHD. Stimulants retain their effectiveness in adolescents (and adults) with symptoms of ADHD. In preschool children, stimulant effect is more variable, and the rate of side effects is higher, especially sadness, irritability, clinging, insomnia, anorexia, and repetitive behaviors (Greenhill et al. 2006). Stimulants can improve attention and reduce excessive distractibility in patients with all three subtypes of ADHD. Many children whose symptoms respond positively to stimulants, however, continue to have deficits such as specific learning disabilities and gaps in knowledge and skills caused by inattention, poor social skills, and family problems. Intensive behavior modification may add to stimulant effect or permit the use of a lower dose of medication, but it is often difficult to implement and sustain behavioral treatment and to transfer improvements from one setting to another. The National Institute of Mental Health (NIMH) Multimodal Treatment of ADHD (MTA) study showed that optimally titrated methylphenidate was more effective for core ADHD symptoms than intensive behavioral therapy, that optimal methylphenidate treatment plus behavioral treatment was more effective than behavioral treatment alone, and

TABLE 8–1. Stimulant preparations

Drug	Formulation	Doses
Methylphenidate		
Generic (IR) (3–4 hours)	Tablet	5, 10, 20
Methylin (IR) (3–4 hours)	Tablet	5, 10, 20[a]
	Chewable tablet	2.5, 5, 10[a]
	Oral solution (grape)	5 mg/5 mL, 10 mg/5 mL
Methylin ER (6–8 hours)	Hydrophilic polymer	10, 20
Ritalin (IR) (3–4 hours)	Tablet	5, 10, 20
Ritalin SR (6–8 hours)	Wax matrix tablet	20
Generic SR (6–8 hours)	Wax matrix tablet	20
Metadate ER (6–8 hours)	Wax matrix tablet	10, 20
Ritalin LA (8–10 hours)	Capsule with beads (sprinkle) Ratio of IR:LA=50:50	10, 20, 30, 40
Metadate CD (6–8 hours)	Capsule Diffucap with beads (sprinkle) 30-pill blister pack or bottle of 100 Ratio of IR:LA=30:70	10, 20, 30, 40, 50, 60
Concerta (12 hours)	Oros (osmotic controlled-release) tablet Ratio of IR:LA=4:14 10% of MPH stays in capsule Maximum FDA-approved dose=72 mg	18, 27, 36, 54 18 mg Oros=5 mg IR bid or tid or 20 mg SR
Daytrana	Transdermal system (patch) Worn for 9 hours for 12-hour duration	10, 15, 20, 30

TABLE 8–1. Stimulant preparations *(continued)*

Drug	Formulation	Doses
Dexmethylphenidate[b]		
Focalin (3–4 hours)	Tablet	2.5, 10
Generic (3–4 hours)	Tablet	2.5, 5, 10
Focalin XR (10–12 hours)	Capsule with beads (sprinkle)	5, 10, 15, 20, 30
	Ratio of IR:LA=50:50	
Dextroamphetamine		
DextroStat (IR) (3–5 hours)	Tablet	5,[a] 10[c]
Dexedrine (IR) (3–5 hours)	Tablet	5
Generic (IR) (3–5 hours)	Tablet	5, 10
LiQUADD (3–5 hours) (dextroamphetamine sulphate)	Oral solution	5 mg/5 mL
Dexedrine Spansule (6–8 hours)	Capsule with beads	5, 10, 15
Dextroamphetamine ER (6–8 hours)	Capsule with beads	5, 10, 15
Lisdexamfetamine dimesylate (Vyvanse) (12–14 hours)	Prodrug (may open capsule—dissolve in water; do not divide capsules)	20, 30, 40, 50, 60, 70

TABLE 8–1. Stimulant preparations *(continued)*

Drug	Formulation	Doses
Mixed salts amphetamine		
Adderall (IR) (3–5 hours)	Tablet	5,[c] 7.5,[c] 10,[c] 12.5,[c] 20,[c] 30[c]
Generic (IR) (3–5 hours)	Tablet	5, 7.5, 10, 12.5, 20, 30
Adderall XR (10–12 hours)	Capsule with beads (sprinkle) Ratio of IR:LA=50:50	5, 10, 15, 20, 25, 30
Generic (XR) (10–12 hours)	Capsule with beads (sprinkle) Ratio of IR:LA=50:50	5, 10, 15, 20, 25, 30

Note. CD=extended-release; ER=extended-release; IR=immediate-release; LA=long-acting; MPH=methylphenidate; SA=short-acting; SR=sustained-release; XR=extended-release.

[a]Scored.
[b]Only the dextro isomer of methylphenidate.
[c]Double-scored.

that any of the MTA treatments were more effective than treatment as usual in the community (mostly stimulants, but at lower doses, fewer doses per day, shorter duration of treatment, and less close monitoring) (MTA Cooperative Group 1999).

When *conduct disorder* or *oppositional defiant disorder* co-exists with ADHD, stimulant medication can reduce defiance, negativism, and impulsive verbal and physical aggression. In children and adolescents with *mental retardation,* stimulants are effective in treating ADHD target symptoms, although effect size is smaller and side effects are more common. Stimulants also reduce symptoms of inattention, impulsivity, and overactivity in some children with *pervasive developmental disorders.*

Boys and adults, with or without ADHD, have similar cognitive and behavioral responses to comparable doses of stimulants, except that children report feeling "funny," whereas adults report euphoria (Donnelly and Rapoport 1985). Stimulants act in the brain by binding to the dopamine transporter, thereby increasing the amount of dopamine available in the synapse. Stimulants may preferentially increase neurotransmitter activity at inhibitory synapses and in inhibitory brain areas. Stimulants are absorbed rapidly from the gut and metabolized rapidly. Stimulant medication effects on ADHD occur primarily as the drug is being absorbed and as the plasma concentration is rising.

There are no useful predictors of whether an individual patient with ADHD will respond to a specific medication. Neurological soft signs, electroencephalogram (EEG), brain scans, or neurochemical measures are not useful predictors of response to stimulants. Although prior studies were mixed, the NIMH MTA study showed that children who have anxiety comorbid with ADHD do not have a reduced response to stimulants. Most patients with ADHD have some positive response to at least one of the stimulant medications, although a substantial number of children respond to one stimulant but not another (Elia et al. 1991). Stimulant effects on individual target symptoms (Table 8–2), however, vary greatly from child to child and even from one symptom to another in a single patient. A given dose may produce improvement in some areas but no change or worsening

TABLE 8–2. Clinical effects of stimulant medications

Motor effects	Reduce activity to level that fits the context
	Decrease excessive talking, noise, and disruption
	Decrease fidgeting and finger-tapping
	Improve handwriting
	Improve fine motor control
Social effects	Reduce off-task behavior
	Improve ability to play and work independently
	Reduce impulsivity
	Decrease intensity of behavior
	Reduce bossiness
	Reduce verbal and physical aggression
	Improve (but not normalize) peer social status
	Reduce noncompliance and defiance with adults
	Improve parent–child interactions
	Parents and teachers respond with less controlling and more positive behavior
Cognitive effects	Improve effort and attention, especially to boring tasks
	Increase on-task behavior
	Reduce distractibility
	Reduce impulsivity
	Increase quantity and accuracy of academic work

in others. Therefore, if one stimulant is ineffective, another should be tried before using another drug class. Methylphenidate is the most commonly used and best-studied stimulant. Amphetamine disadvantages include negative attitudes of pharmacists and higher potential for abuse. Compared with methylphenidate, amphetamine may have a slightly greater incidence of side effects such as growth retardation, appetite suppression, and compulsive behaviors.

Dexmethylphenidate (Focalin) contains only the dextro isomer of methylphenidate. Compared with conventional d,l methylphenidate, half the dose of dexmethylphenidate appears to be just as effective, with fewer side effects, and perhaps longer duration. Longer-acting stimulant preparations are now most commonly used. They are especially appealing for children in whom the duration of action of the standard formulations is very short (2.5–3.0 hours); when severe rebound occurs; or when administering medication every 4 hours (or at school) is inconvenient, inconsistent, stigmatizing, impossible, or insufficiently supervised to prevent diversion of the drug. The many different formulations of methylphenidate and amphetamine are useful in tailoring treatment to each patient (see Table 8–1).

Although short-term efficacy of stimulants has been clearly demonstrated, it is much more difficult to demonstrate long-term effects. Existing studies have had methodological problems (e.g., naturalistic treatment assignment; comorbidity; premature termination of drug; doses too high, too low, or poorly timed; inconsistent adherence to medication; individual variation in response; and insensitive outcome instruments). A long-term prospective randomized controlled trial assigning children with ADHD to stimulant medication or placebo or other treatment is neither ethical nor feasible.

Initiation and Ongoing Treatment

The decision to medicate a child with ADHD is based on the child's inattention, impulsivity, and often hyperactivity that are not due to another treatable cause and that are persistent and severe enough to cause functional impairment at school and usually at home and with peers. For safety reasons, parents must be willing to monitor the medication and to attend appointments with the child. An important part of treatment is education of the child, family, and teacher, including explicitly debunking common myths about stimulant treatment. Stimulants do *not* have a paradoxical sedative action, do *not* lead to drug abuse, and *do* continue to be effective after puberty.

Multiple outcome measures that use more than one source and setting are essential. The clinician obtains baseline data from the school on behavior and academic performance before initiating stimulant medication. The physician should work closely with parents on adjusting the size and timing of doses and obtain frequent reports from teachers and annual academic testing. The Child Attention Problems (CAP) Rating Scale (see Tables 3–3 and 3–4) or the IOWA Conners Scale (see Chapter 3) is useful in gathering weekly data from teachers.

Many experts recommend a systematic stimulant titration using the full range of doses—for example, 5, 10, 15, and 20 mg of methylphenidate (highest dose omitted for very young or small children). Body weight serves only as a rough guide. Doses of amphetamine or dexmethylphenidate (Focalin) are half the milligrams of methylphenidate. A strategy that is preferred by many clinicians and parents is to start stimulant medication at a low dose and increase by half (if necessary and if pill is scored) or whole pills (within the usual recommended range) every week or two, monitoring response (ideally including teacher ratings) and side effects. By age 3 years, children's absorption, distribution, protein binding, and metabolism of stimulants are similar to those of an adult, although adults may have more side effects than do children at the same milligram per kilogram of body weight dose.

The onset of clinical effect for immediate-release methylphenidate and amphetamine is within 30 minutes after each dose. A single dose is usually effective for 3–4 hours. Of the immediate-release forms, amphetamine typically has a longer therapeutic duration than methylphenidate. A typical regimen for the immediate-release preparations would be thrice-daily dosing, with medication given after breakfast, after lunch, and after school. Starting with only a morning dose may be useful in assessing drug effect, by comparing morning and afternoon school performance. The need for an after-school dose or for medication on weekends is individually determined by considering target symptoms. A third dose after school has been shown to improve behavior without increasing sleep problems (Kent et al. 1995). Most children with moderate or severe symptoms of ADHD need full coverage, all day and all week. The long-acting formulations are typically given once a day, in the morning, with supplementation with immediate release if necessary.

If the initial stimulant drug choice is not effective or not well tolerated, more than half of nonresponders to methylphenidate or amphetamine respond to the other stimulant.

Medical monitoring includes, at a minimum, pulse rate and blood pressure initially and at times of dose change; weight at baseline, during titration, and two to three times a year; and height at baseline and then several times a year. Prior to prescribing stimulant medication, the clinician should take a cardiac history, including any patient structural abnormalities, chest pain, palpitations, fainting, and reduced exercise tolerance and family history of arrhythmias, early cardiac death, or sudden unexplained death. Electrocardiogram (ECG) monitoring prior to and during stimulant treatment has been controversial. Following the FDA warnings in 2006 regarding sudden death in patients with structural cardiac abnormalities or other serious heart problems, the American Heart Association issued a statement in 2008 that recommended obtaining an ECG prior to stimulant treatment. This recommendation lacked specific supporting evidence, and later the same year the American Academy of Pediatrics (supported by the American Academy of Child and Adolescent Psychiatry) issued a statement (Perrin et al. 2008) concluding that routine pretreatment cardiac tests are *not* currently indicated unless there is known/suspected cardiac disorder or symptoms. If there are such findings on history or pediatric examination, an ECG and often a pediatric cardiology consultation are indicated. The clinician should look for and inquire about tics at baseline and at every visit. Periodic reevaluation of the need for a dosage increase or decrease or change in timing of administration will optimize improvement.

Although pharmacological tolerance has been reported occasionally, medication administration is often irregular, and lack of adherence should be considered when medication appears to become ineffective. The child should not be responsible for his or her own medication, because these youngsters are impulsive and forgetful at best, and most dislike the idea of taking medication, even when they can verbalize its positive effects and report few if any side effects. They will often avoid, "forget," surreptitiously spit out, or simply refuse to take a dose of medication. Apparent decreased drug effect may be caused by a reaction to a stressful change at home or school, lower efficacy of a generic preparation, or abatement of an initial positive placebo effect. If tolerance does occur, the other stimulant may be substituted.

The duration of medication treatment is individually determined by whether drug-responsive target symptoms are still present. Treatment may be required through adolescence and into adulthood. If behavioral symptoms are not severe outside of the school setting, the young person may have an annual drug-free trial of at least 2 weeks, or even the whole summer if symptoms are mild. If school behavior and academic performance are stable, a carefully monitored trial off medication during the school year (but *not* at the beginning) will provide data on whether medication is still needed.

Risks and Side Effects

Most side effects are similar for all stimulants (Table 8–3). Giving medication after meals reduces appetite suppression. Insomnia may be due to ADHD symptoms, oppositional refusal to go to bed, separation anxiety, or stimulant effect or rebound. Preexisting sleep problems are common in patients with ADHD. Stimulants may either worsen or improve irritable mood. Other than mildly elevated blood pressure, cardiovascular side effects are exceedingly rare. Toxic effects may result if a child chews one of the long-acting forms instead of swallowing it.

The use of stimulants in patients with a personal or family history of tics has been controversial because of concern that new, persistent tics might be precipitated, especially in those children who are at genetic risk. The physician must balance the impairment resulting from tics with that from ADHD symptoms, considering the efficacy and side-effect profile of alternative medications. With appropriate informed consent and careful clinical monitoring, a stimulant (methylphenidate) may remain the first choice. Tics are extremely common in children with ADHD, with or without stimulant medication, and tend to wax and wane. Several studies have demonstrated that few children develop new or worsened tics while on methylphenidate, and many preexisting tics are unchanged or

TABLE 8–3.   Side effects of stimulant medications

**Common side effects
(try dose reduction)**

Anorexia
Weight loss or slowed weight gain (may be worse with amphetamine)
Irritability (may be worse with amphetamine)
Abdominal pain
Headaches
Easy crying

Less common side effects

Mildly elevated blood pressure
Insomnia (may be worse with amphetamine)
Dysphoria (may be worse with amphetamine)
Social withdrawal
Impaired cognitive test performance (especially at very high dosages)
Decrease in expected weight gain
Rebound overactivity and irritability (try adding small afternoon or evening dose)
Habits such as skin picking and nail biting
Allergic rash, hives, or conjunctivitis
Transient motor tics (may be worse with amphetamine)

Infrequent side effects

Dizziness
Nausea
Anxiety and fearfulness
Stuttering

TABLE 8–3. Side effects of stimulant medications *(continued)*

Rare but potentially serious side effects (usually reversible)	Exacerbation or precipitation of tics (may be worse with amphetamine)
	Depression
	Growth retardation
	Tachycardia
	Hypertension
	Psychosis with hallucinations
	Stereotyped activities or compulsions
Reported with Concerta only	Capsule lodged in throat
Side effects reported with Daytrana only	Skin irritation under patch
	Allergy to methylphenidate

Source. Adapted from Efron et al. 1997.

even improve (Bloch et al. 2009). There is some evidence that high doses of amphetamine can increase tic severity, which may persist (Kurlan 2002).

Although stimulant-induced growth retardation has been a concern, and weight and height should be monitored, any decreases in expected weight gain and growth are small and rarely clinically significant (Faraone et al. 2008). The magnitude may be dose related and may be greater with dextroamphetamine than with methylphenidate. Attenuation of effect has been reported. Medication-free summers (if clinically appropriate) may facilitate height or weight normalization.

Rebound effects such as increased excitability, activity, talkativeness, irritability, and insomnia, beginning 3–15 hours after a dose, may be seen as each dose or the last dose of the day wears off or for up to several days after sudden withdrawal of high daily doses of stimulants. These effects may resemble a worsening of the original symptoms. Management strategies include increasing structure after school, giving a dose of medication in the afternoon that is smaller than the midday dose, or using a long-acting formulation. If the rebound effect is severe, an alternate agent (atomoxetine, guanfacine, or clonidine) can be added to or substituted for the stimulant.

Clinically relevant contraindications to the use of stimulant medication are schizophrenia or other acute psychosis, glaucoma, or recent stimulant drug abuse. When potential abuse of stimulant medication by the patient, or, more often, by peers or family members is a concern, Concerta may be a good choice, as its once a day administration is easier to supervise, and the physical characteristics of the pill (methylphenidate mixed with an osmotic "sponge") make it impossible to crush and snort or inject. Vyvanse is also not abusable, because of the need for cleavage of the amino acid before the amphetamine is active.

No evidence indicates that stimulants as clinically prescribed decrease the seizure threshold or precipitate bipolar disorder.

A selective serotonin reuptake inhibitor (SSRI) may be added to a stimulant for the treatment of comorbid ADHD and depression or anxiety (for symptoms remaining after stimulant treatment).

Stimulants are used in combination with atomoxetine, clonidine, or guanfacine to treat symptoms resistant to a stimulant alone. This is theoretically appealing because of complementary actions and non-overlapping side-effect profiles.

■ ATOMOXETINE

Atomoxetine (Strattera) is a potent inhibitor of presynaptic norepinephrine transporters with minimal affinity for other receptors or transporters.

Indications and Efficacy

Atomoxetine is the first nonstimulant approved by the FDA for the treatment of ADHD. Randomized controlled trials have shown efficacy in inattentive and hyperactive-impulsive symptoms of ADHD in preschoolers through adolescents as reported by parents and teachers (Kelsey et al. 2004; Michelson et al. 2001). Atomoxetine is effective in some youth who have not responded to stimulant treatment. In trials, about half of subjects are atomoxetine responders (Newcorn et al. 2009). In responders, the effect size is somewhat lower than that typically seen with stimulants. Atomoxetine improves comorbid oppositional symptoms (improvement greater at higher doses) (Newcorn et al. 2005) and comorbid anxiety symptoms. In addition to a different side-effect profile, which is useful for patients who do not tolerate stimulants, atomoxetine provides 24-hour coverage, which is especially helpful with the evening and early morning symptoms not covered by stimulants. Atomoxetine might be the first choice for patients with ADHD if stimulants are refused or not feasible (controlled substances) or for patients with preexisting severe behavior problems before school, insomnia, or low weight.

Initiation and Ongoing Treatment

Atomoxetine may be given once a day (morning or evening) or divided into two doses (with breakfast and dinner) to reduce side effects. The starting dose is 0.3 mg/kg/day (usually in a single daily dose) for a week, then increased over 1–3 weeks to an initial target dose of 1.2 mg/kg/day. The FDA maximum dose is 1.4 mg/kg/day or 100 mg, whichever is less, but the off-label maximum dose (demonstrated safe in clinical trials) is 1.8 mg/kg/day. The maximum response on a particular dose may be delayed several weeks or even months, requiring patience (especially when compared to the immediate effects of the stimulants). Tapering is not required when discontinuing this medicine. Atomoxetine is metabolized via the CYP2D6 pathway. Some patients are poor metabolizers due to genetic makeup or drug interactions, but there are not adverse clinical consequences and genotyping is not recommended.

Atomoxetine may be combined with a stimulant in patients partially responsive to each.

Risks and Side Effects

Side effects are generally mild and include sedation, decreased appetite, nausea, abdominal pain, and dizziness. Taking the medication with food improves tolerability. There are slight increases in blood pressure and pulse (rarely clinically significant), but no QTc prolongation on ECG. Atomoxetine may offer the advantages of desipramine without the risk of cardiac side effects or danger in overdose. Atomoxetine does not increase tics (Allen et al. 2006) or lower the seizure threshold. The capsules must not be opened, as the contents are caustic to the eye. Rare side effects include syncope, vomiting, constipation, irritability, and (in the presence of comorbid bipolar disorder) manic activation. Atomoxetine has two FDA bolded warnings: one regarding extremely rare severe liver injury and one (based on weak evidence) of increased hostility and aggression or suicidal ideation. Routine liver function monitoring is not recommended, but parents should be instructed that if jaundice, unexplained abdominal symptoms, pruritus, or dark urine appear, the medication should be stopped and the physician should be called so that liver function tests can be obtained. Atomoxetine does not have a physiological withdrawal syndrome if stopped suddenly, although symptoms of ADHD are likely to return.

■ GUANFACINE AND CLONIDINE

Guanfacine hydrochloride and clonidine are α-adrenergic agonists developed for the treatment of hypertension. They had been used as second- or third-line treatments for ADHD, despite relatively sparse supporting research. Recently developed extended-release formulations of guanfacine (Intuniv) (once a day) and clonidine (Kapvay) (twice a day) have been studied in randomized controlled trials and given FDA indications for the treatment of ADHD. Kapvay also has a specific indication as an add-on to stimulant therapy for ADHD. These longer-acting formulations have more research to support their use, and they avoid daily rebound of symptoms or gaps in effectiveness and the inconvenience of needing to be given three or four times a day. Also, like atomoxetine, they provide coverage for symptoms of ADHD in the early morning and the evening, when stimulants are not active. Comparing the two drugs, in general, guanfacine has more evidence for treatment effect in inattention, and clonidine is more sedating.

Indications and Efficacy

Attention-Deficit/Hyperactivity Disorder

Clonidine improves frustration tolerance and compliance and reduces emotional outbursts in ADHD. It may be used at bedtime to decrease ADHD overarousal or oppositional behavior or to ameliorate insomnia caused by stimulant effect or rebound.

In a study comparing immediate-release methylphenidate and clonidine, the combination, and placebo, methylphenidate was most effective by teacher report and class observation, with the fewest adverse effects of the active treatments. Clonidine was less effective for ADHD symptoms and caused sedation, but showed improvement on parent ratings. The combination showed little evidence of added benefit and no increase in side effects (Palumbo et al. 2008). A small randomized controlled trial comparing immediate-release methylphenidate and clonidine and the combination in youth with ADHD plus aggressive oppositional or conduct symptoms found that all three treatment conditions were associated with significant improvement in attention, impulsivity, and oppositional and conduct symptoms on parent and teacher rating scales and laboratory measures, with few differences among groups. There were no safety findings related to the combination (Connor et al. 2000).

A randomized controlled trial (Jain et al. 2011) of two doses of extended-release clonidine (0.2 mg/day and 0.4 mg/day) versus placebo in children with hyperactive/impulsive or combined type ADHD found parent report of efficacy of both doses, starting at 2 weeks after the target dose was reached.

Two randomized placebo-controlled trials have demonstrated efficacy of extended-release guanfacine as monotherapy for both hyperactive/impulsive and inattentive symptoms of ADHD as well as for oppositional symptoms by parent, teacher, and clinician ratings (Biederman et al. 2008; Sallee et al. 2009). Extended-release guanfacine has also been shown to be effective for symptoms of ADHD when added to stimulant medication, in stimulant partial responders (Wilens et al. 2010).

Tourette's Disorder

A modest randomized controlled trial of children with tic disorders and ADHD showed that guanfacine (immediate release) significantly improved (compared with placebo) teacher and clinician ratings of ADHD symptoms, led to decreased errors on a continuous performance test (while placebo subjects increased errors), and decreased tic severity by 31% (compared with 0% on placebo) (Scahill et al. 2001).

The efficacy of clonidine for Tourette's disorder per se has been controversial. However a randomized controlled trial in children with both chronic tics and ADHD showed efficacy of clonidine in reducing both tics and impulsivity/hyperactivity (Tourette's Syndrome Study Group 2002).

Other Symptoms

Guanfacine or clonidine may be useful in the management of aggressive behavior, impulsivity, oppositional behavior, self-injurious behavior, and agitation in a variety of conditions, including PTSD and mental retardation.

Initiation and Ongoing Treatment

Before guanfacine or clonidine is initiated, a cardiovascular history and a physical examination (including blood pressure and pulse rate) are needed. An ECG may be advisable for preschool children, although the American Heart Association guidelines do not mandate ECG monitoring with these drugs. If there is a family history of diabetes or clinical indications in the patient, a fasting blood glucose may be indicated. These drugs are contraindicated in patients with a history of syncope, bradycardia, or heart block.

One mg of guanfacine is equivalent to 0.1 mg of clonidine. One of these α-adrenergic agonists can be switched to the other by a gradual cross-taper.

Immediate-release guanfacine is started at 0.5 mg/day and then gradually increased by 0.5 mg every 3–4 days to a maximum daily dose of 4 mg in three divided doses. Intuniv is titrated from 1 mg/day, increasing by 1 mg/day each week to a maximum of 4 mg/day. The target dose is 0.05–0.08 mg/kg/day. The maximum dose is 4 mg/day or 0.12 mg/kg/day, whichever is less. It is not mg-to-mg equivalent with immediate-release guanfacine. Discontinuation should be by gradual taper.

Immediate-release clonidine is started at a low dose of 0.05 mg/day at bedtime and titrated gradually over 2–4 weeks to 0.15–0.40 mg/day (0.003–0.01 mg/kg/day) in four divided doses (for immediate release), in order to minimize sedation. The medication should be continued for 2–8 weeks at the maximal dose before determining effectiveness (Pliszka et al. 2000). Clonidine is available in a transdermal skin patch that may improve ability to administer medication as prescribed and may reduce effects on blood pressure by smoothing blood levels. The transdermal form is effective for only 4–5 days in children, compared with 7 days in adults; the patch may be cut to adjust the dose (Hunt 1987). Clonidine extended-release is started at 0.1 mg/day in two divided doses and increased by 0.1 mg/day each week to a target of 0.4 mg/day, divided into every-12-hour doses. Doses of immediate- and extended-release clonidine are not mg-for-mg equivalent. Any form of clonidine should be discontinued by gradual tapering to avoid withdrawal tachycardia, hypertension, headache, and nausea.

Risks and Side Effects

The extended-release forms must not be crushed, chewed, or broken.

Guanfacine has fewer and milder side effects (primarily irritability, sedation, headache, and abdominal pain) and less rebound than clonidine. Surprisingly, guanfacine used for the treatment of ADHD has little effect on pulse or blood pressure, although syncope has been reported rarely in patients with ADHD or Tourette's disorder.

The most troublesome side effect of clonidine is somnolence, which is most prominent early in treatment and generally decreases after 4–8 weeks. Patients may experience daily rebound hyperactivity and irritability or insomnia when the immediate release form is used. The extended-release formulation of clonidine may produce less somnolence and rebound. The most serious potential adverse effects of clonidine are cardiovascular and include hypotension, bradycardia, rebound tachycardia and hypertension, and asymptomatic ECG conduction changes. Clonidine may worsen symptoms of dysphoria. Less common side effects include headache, abdominal pain, irritability, nightmares, rash, and decreased glucose tolerance. The skin patch often causes a local hypersensitivity reaction.

In the past, anecdotal reports of sudden death in children who at one time had been taking both methylphenidate and clonidine generated some concern, but evidence linking the drugs to the deaths is tenuous (Wilens and Spencer 1999). Pending further clarification, extra caution has been advised when treating preschoolers, children with cardiac disease, when combining clonidine with additional medications, or when adherence to consistent medication administration is uncertain.

■ ANTIDEPRESSANTS

Medications called *antidepressants* that are commonly used for the treatment of a variety of disorders in children and adolescents are listed in Table 8–4. Evidence related to their pediatric use is growing, although more research is needed, particularly studies comparing drugs of the same class. Interestingly, despite the name of the drug class, in children and adolescents, evidence is stronger for benefit in anxiety disorders than in depression. The safest and most commonly used class of antidepressants is the selective serotonin reuptake inhibitors (SSRIs), which include citalopram (Celexa), escitalopram (Lexapro), fluoxetine (Prozac), fluvoxamine (Luvox), paroxetine (Paxil), and sertraline (Zoloft).

Bupropion (Wellbutrin) has a novel chemical structure and inhibits norepinephrine and dopamine. It is available in immediate- and sustained- and extended-release forms. Because of the side effect of increased seizure risk (likely dose-related), bupropion is contraindicated in youth with epilepsy, eating disorders, or other risk factors for seizures. Currently, empirical support exists for its use in ADHD, but not pediatric depression.

Mirtazapine (Remeron) is unique in its noradrenergic and specific serotonergic mechanisms. Although generally well tolerated, weight gain can occur. Although it is FDA-approved for depression in adults, evidence does not support efficacy in pediatric major depression. A recent open-label pilot study explored the use of mirtazapine in youth with social phobia (Mrakotsky et al. 2008).

Duloxetine (Cymbalta) has FDA approval for use in treating depression and generalized anxiety disorder in adults; however, it has not been studied in youth. Case reports suggest it may be beneficial in adolescents with pain and depression (Meighen 2007).

Several atypical antidepressants have empirical support in adults but not in youth. Trazodone (Desyrel), a serotonin reuptake inhibitor and a mixed serotonergic agonist and antagonist, has been used for insomnia in children. Its use in boys is very limited because of the potentially serious side effect of priapism (prolonged painful erection of the penis). Venlafaxine (Effexor) is a potent inhibitor of

TABLE 8–4. Antidepressant medications most often used in children and adolescents

Generic name	Brand name	Typical[a] daily dose <18 years	Indications supported by RCT <18 years
Selective serotonin reuptake inhibitors			
Citalopram	Celexa	20–60 mg	Depression
Escitalopram	Lexapro	10–20 mg	Depression
Fluoxetine	Prozac	5–40 mg	Depression, social phobia, GAD,
		10–60 mg	OCD
Fluvoxamine	Luvox	100–200 mg	OCD, social phobia, SAD, GAD
Sertraline	Zoloft	25–250 mg	OCD
		25–200 mg	GAD, depression
Bupropion	Wellbutrin	100–300 mg	ADHD
	Wellbutrin SR		
Tricyclic antidepressants[b]			
Clomipramine	Anafranil	50–200 mg	OCD
		1–3 mg/kg	

Note. ADHD=attention-deficit/hyperactivity disorder; GAD=generalized anxiety disorder; OCD=obsessive-compulsive disorder; RCT=randomized controlled trial; SAD=separation anxiety disorder.

[a]Starting doses are lower. Within this range, children require lower doses than do adolescents.
[b]Divided doses required for children.

serotonin and norepinephrine reuptake and a weak inhibitor of dopamine uptake. Its problematic side-effect profile in youth has led to high dropout rates in clinical trials. Venlafaxine seems to be more beneficial in anxiety treatment than depression in youth. Expert consensus places it as a third-line option for treatment of resistant pediatric major depression along with bupropion, mirtazapine, and duloxetine (Hughes et al. 2007). Despite demonstrated efficacy in pediatric ADHD, anxiety disorders, and enuresis (but not pediatric depression), tricyclic antidepressants (TCAs) are very rarely used in youth, because of their problematic side-effect profile, including cardiac effects that require ECG monitoring and lethality in overdose. For each of the indications, safer and generally equally or more effective drugs are available.

Indications and Efficacy

Depression

SSRIs are the first-line medication treatment for youth with depression. In addition to inhibition of serotonin reuptake, longer-term treatment also generally results in down regulation of serotonin receptors and also modulates transmission of serotonin. Some of the SSRIs also have additional pharmacological mechanisms.

The FDA has approved pediatric indications in major depressive disorder (MDD) for fluoxetine (age 8 years and older) and escitalopram (age 12 years and older). Fluoxetine has the best-documented efficacy from randomized controlled trials. Paroxetine is rarely used, because of mixed evidence on efficacy and concern about side effects in youth. The results of two studies of sertraline (reported as one merged study) support efficacy in depressed youth. The extremely high "placebo response" (more accurately described as nonspecific positive response to being in a clinical trial) has made it difficult to demonstrate superiority of antidepressants to placebo in pediatric depression. Data from citalopram trials are inconsistent, and fluvoxamine has not been studied in pediatric depression.

Research evidence is lacking with regard to comparative effectiveness among the SSRIs, so choice is based on target symptoms, comorbidity, side effects, half-life, interactions with other medications, positive familial experience with or response to the agent, patient/family preference, or a trial of the drug in the particular patient. For example, fluoxetine's long half-life may be an advantage if missed doses are likely, but side effects or drug–drug interactions can persist for weeks after fluoxetine is discontinued, and fine-tuning of the dose may be difficult. If a patient does not respond well to the first one chosen, a trial with another SSRI is typically indicated. A Treatment of Resistant Depression in Adolescents (TORDIA) randomized controlled trial found that in teens with MDD or dysthymia who had failed to respond to an adequate trial of an SSRI, a medication change with added cognitive-behavioral therapy (CBT) was better than switching medications alone. Switching to fluoxetine or citalopram was as effective as switching to venlafaxine, and venlafaxine produced more side effects (Brent et al. 2008).

Efforts should be made to treat to full remission of symptoms. After a child or adolescent has been asymptomatic for 6–12 months, the clinician may consider slowly tapering the medication. Timing of a discontinuation trial should avoid stressful life events or predictably difficult times such as a new school year. Extrapolating from adult data, it is recommended that youth with multiple depressive episodes continue maintenance medication indefinitely.

Obsessive-Compulsive Disorder

Multiple SSRIs, including fluoxetine, fluvoxamine, paroxetine, and sertraline, have been shown in randomized controlled trials to be efficacious in the treatment of OCD in youth. Drugs with FDA indications for OCD in children and adolescents are sertraline (age 6 years and older), fluoxetine (7 years and older), fluvoxamine (8 years and older), and the tricyclic clomipramine (10 years and older), a third-line choice due to safety and tolerability issues. Clomipramine is generally reserved for use as an augmentation strategy to an SSRI, and is less commonly used for this purpose than are atypical antipsychotics.

School Avoidance or Separation Anxiety Disorder

Fluvoxamine has been shown to be more effective than placebo in studies of youth with social phobia, separation anxiety disorder (SAD), or generalized anxiety disorder (GAD) (Walkup et al. 2001). In a large study of youth with SAD, GAD, or social phobia, sertraline was superior to placebo; sertraline plus CBT demonstrated an even stronger response (Walkup et al. 2008). Therefore, the first-choice medication for treating these disorders is an SSRI, although medication is considered to be one component of a multimodal treatment plan and is recommended only when symptoms are moderate to severe with significant functional impairment. Some clinicians add a benzodiazepine to SSRI treatment for a very short time, as a bridge in cases with severe symptoms, until the SSRI is effective.

Other Anxiety Disorders

A multisite randomized controlled trial by the Research Units on Pediatric Psychopharmacology Anxiety Study Group has demonstrated efficacy of fluvoxamine in children and adolescents with social phobia, SAD, or GAD (Walkup et al. 2001). Sertraline was efficacious in a small randomized controlled trial for GAD in children and adolescents (Rynn et al. 2001).

Consensus among experts is that there is no evidence that one SSRI is more effective than another for pediatric anxiety disorders. In a large randomized controlled study of 7–17-year-olds with SAD, GAD, or social phobia, combination treatment (CBT plus sertraline) was more effective than either monotherapy or placebo, and each active treatment as monotherapy (SBT or sertraline) was significantly superior to placebo (Walkup et al. 2008). Fluoxetine was shown to be effective for youth with GAD and social phobia, but not for SAD (Birmaher et al. 2003). In another study, Wagner et al. (2004) found youth with social anxiety to respond favorably to paroxetine. A large randomized controlled trial in youth with social anxiety disorder found venlafaxine extended release (ER) to be superior in efficacy to placebo (March et al. 2007).

The efficacy of fluoxetine in selective mutism is suggested by one small controlled trial (although most subjects had remaining symptoms) (Black and Uhde 1994) and open trials. Despite the lack of research, SSRIs are sometimes used to treat panic disorder in youth, based on extrapolation from adults.

Attention-Deficit/Hyperactivity Disorder

Bupropion has been shown to be effective in both children and adults with ADHD, with an effect size equivalent to methylphenidate (Barrickman et al. 1995).

TCAs, especially imipramine and desipramine, have demonstrated efficacy in the treatment of ADHD. Now that a variety of safer alternative drugs (stimulants in many formulations, atomoxetine, guanfacine, clonidine) have demonstrated efficacy in ADHD, TCAs (most often nortriptyline) would be a fourth- or fifth-line choice for the treatment of ADHD, used only if other drugs are ineffective or not tolerated.

Pervasive Developmental Disorders

There is some evidence that the SSRIs such as fluoxetine (Hollander et al. 2005) may be useful in reducing aggression, temper problems, self-injurious behavior, and stereotyped behavior. The results of a more recent trial of citalopram for repetitive behaviors in children with autism were disappointing (King et al. 2009). The atypical antipsychotics are now more commonly used to treat severe irritability or aggression in youth with autism.

Enuresis

Enuresis can be addressed by the child's primary care physician, or in a multimodal treatment program that addresses the common medical contributing factors and implements behavioral strategies. Imipramine has been replaced by desmopressin (DDAVP) as the first-choice drug used in the treatment of enuresis.

Initiation and Ongoing Treatment

Typical therapeutic daily dose ranges are listed in Table 8–4. The general principle "start low and go slow" applies.

Selective Serotonin Reuptake Inhibitors

SSRIs do not require medical assessment prior to or during treatment other than pregnancy testing for menstruating females at risk for pregnancy. Particularly with anxiety disorders, very low initial doses and slow titration will minimize side effects that could lead to refusal to take medication. A useful starting strategy is to prescribe the lowest dose pill available, or half a pill, if scored. The liquid formulation of fluoxetine may be used for very gradual titration. Fluoxetine is sometimes prescribed on an every-other-day basis because it has a long half-life and active metabolites. A very long-acting form (Prozac Weekly) is now available for patients who may be nonadherent with daily medication, once a therapeutic dose is found and tolerability in that patient is established.

Bupropion

The clinical history should include queries regarding seizures and factors that predispose to seizures (e.g., head trauma, other central nervous system problems, other drugs that lower the seizure threshold, eating disorders). An EEG may be indicated before starting bupropion if a seizure diathesis is possible. Bupropion is administered in two or three daily doses, beginning with a dose of 37.5 or 50 mg twice a day, with gradual titration over 2 weeks to a usual maximum of 250 mg/day (300–400 mg/day in adolescents). A single dose should not exceed 150 mg. Blood levels do not appear to be useful. Longer-acting sustained SR, XR, and XL formulations are now available that may be given once or twice a day.

Risks and Side Effects

Selective Serotonin Reuptake Inhibitors

Most side effects are mild, emerge early in treatment, and resolve over time. Low starting doses and slow, gradual titration can limit the development of adverse effects. Common somatic side effects include headaches, anorexia, weight loss, weight gain, bruxism, nausea, tremors, drowsiness, and vivid or strange dreams. Increased activity levels can occur, perhaps related in part to akathisia. Symptoms of behavioral activation include restlessness, insomnia, social disinhibition, and agitation or aggression. Bipolar switching or manic reaction is a less common but potentially serious adverse effect to any antidepressant, and can include changes in mood, sleep, behavior, and impulse control. All antidepressant medications, including SSRIs, have an FDA "black box warning" regarding risk of increased suicidal thoughts and behaviors. Although the increased risk is small, careful monitoring is necessary, especially as medication is started and following dose adjustments. In reported studies, children who reported new or increased suicidal thoughts or behaviors typically had preexisting risk factors. Some patients develop apathy or an amotivational syndrome after weeks or months of SSRI treatment, consisting of emotional blunting, decreased motivation, passivity, and loss of interest and energy. This can superficially resemble sedation or worsening of depression, and parents and patients may not identify the cause. A small decrease in dose may be helpful. Pediatric clinicians are not used to considering sexual side effects, but the sexual dysfunction commonly associated with SSRIs (decreased libido, anorgasmia, and erectile dysfunction) may be distressing for adolescents. Bleeding or bruising is very rare but possible (Lake et al. 2000).

Because SSRIs inhibit the cytochrome P450 isoenzymes, there is considerable potential for adverse drug interactions. Serotonin syndrome is a very rare, potentially fatal reaction to the addition or increase in dose of a serotonergic agent (most often in combination with another prescribed or over-the-counter medication or an herbal remedy) characterized by extreme restlessness, agitation, fever, myoclonic jerking movements, severe hyperreflexia, clonus, fasciculation, nausea, vomiting, and diarrhea. Seizures, severe hypotension, ventricular tachycardia, and disseminated intravascular coagulation can occur in severe cases. Deaths have been reported with large ingestions of SSRIs.

Withdrawal symptoms, including dizziness, headache, chills, tiredness, nausea, vomiting, and diarrhea, may occur after sudden discontinuation of an SSRI. This is less of a problem with fluoxetine, because of its very long half-life, and is more likely with paroxetine and fluvoxamine. Mild withdrawal symptoms can occur even with missed doses in some youth. Citalopram and escitalopram have few significant drug interactions because of their weak hepatic cytochrome P450 enzyme inhibition, and they are good options in patients who are on multiple medications. Fluoxetine's long half-life reduces the risk of discontinuation withdrawal symptoms, but the extensive washout period required complicates a subsequent medication trial, if switching drugs is necessary. Among SSRIs, fluvoxamine likely has the lowest incidence of sexual side effects, but sleep disturbances can be a problem. Paroxetine requires exact adherence and slow taper if discontinued, due to its shorter half-life and increased risk for withdrawal symptoms.

Bupropion

Common adverse effects include irritability, insomnia, anorexia, and tic exacerbations. Less commonly, edema, rashes, and nocturia have been reported. Increased seizure risk was discussed above.

■ LITHIUM CARBONATE

Lithium carbonate, a naturally occurring salt, is the most-studied mood stabilizer for children and adolescents. It is FDA-approved for the treatment of mania in patients age 12 and older.

Indications and Efficacy

Mood Disorder

Lithium may be considered in the treatment of bipolar affective disorder, mixed or manic, and for prophylaxis of bipolar disorder in children and adolescents who have a documented history of recurrent episodes. It is effective for acute stabilization in many adolescents with mania, although adjunctive antipsychotic medication or a benzodiazepine (e.g., lorazepam) is often required. Children and adolescents with mania tend to have a less dramatic response to lithium than do adults. Mania in children with preadolescent onset tends to have a poorer response to lithium than does adolescent-onset mania (Strober et al. 1988).

Aggression

Several small studies of youth with severe aggression, especially with impulsivity and explosive affect, showed lithium to be effective in reducing aggression, hostility, and tantrums. Lithium may be useful in intellectually disabled youth with severe aggression directed toward themselves or others.

Initiation and Ongoing Treatment

Lithium should not be prescribed unless the family is willing and able to consistently administer multiple daily doses and obtain lithium blood levels. In addition to the usual medical history and physical examination, complete blood count (CBC) with differential, electrolytes, thyroid function studies, blood urea nitrogen (BUN), and creatinine should be determined before lithium is started. A urinalysis and ECG also should be obtained. An EEG may be indicated. Sexually active adolescent girls should have a pregnancy test.

     Lithium carbonate is the most commonly used formulation because of its reliable serum levels and reasonable cost. Controlled-release lithium (Lithobid, 300 mg, or Eskalith CR, 450 mg) may be used, especially in younger children. Because these formulations are not cleared as rapidly as regular lithium, twice-daily administration is sufficient, and more steady blood levels are achieved. Lithium citrate is available as an oral solution (300 mg lithium per 5 mL). No systematic studies have been done in children to compare the efficacy and side effects of different dosing schedules.

In prepubertal children, traditional practice is to start lithium at 300 mg/day for several weeks and slowly increase it to 900 mg/day in divided doses. Usual child and adolescent therapeutic doses range from 900 to 1,200 mg/day, although daily doses of up to 2,000 mg may be required. Therapeutic levels can be safely attained in a much shorter time by using a weight-based dosage guide (Weller et al. 1986). Also, published nomograms can be used to calculate dosages based on blood levels after single test doses (Alessi et al. 1994; Geller and Fetner 1989). The higher glomerular filtration rate in children compared with adults usually requires a higher milligram-per-kilogram dose before puberty. A weight-based pediatric titration strategy starts with 15–20 mg/kg/day in two or three divided doses. Dose is increased by 300 mg every 4–5 days, based on clinical response, side effects, and serum levels.

Lithium's half-life could permit once-a-day dosing in adolescents. However, because children have more rapid lithium clearance than do adults, multiple divided doses may be necessary to maintain therapeutic levels. In addition, some patients have gastrointestinal distress when they take the entire daily dose at bedtime. Lithium is therefore usually given two or three times a day with meals, even though divided doses have the disadvantage of potentially decreasing adherence to the prescribed regimen.

Therapeutic levels in children are generally similar to those in adults: 0.6–1.2 mEq/L. Under usual circumstances, levels should not exceed 1.4 mEq/L. Peak serum levels will occur within 1–2 hours after ingestion. Steady-state serum levels are achieved after 5 days. To measure the serum level, blood should be drawn 8–12 hours after the last evening dose and before the first morning dose. Levels are obtained once or twice weekly during the initial dosage adjustment and monthly thereafter.

The clinician should periodically check BUN and creatinine or creatinine clearance because lithium may alter kidney function. A thyroid-stimulating hormone (TSH) test should be obtained every 4–6 months. The clinician must be alert to possible clinical signs of hypothyroidism that could be mistaken for fatigue or a retarded depression.

No studies have addressed the issue of how long to continue lithium. A naturalistic study (Strober et al. 1990) found that adolescents who discontinued lithium were three times more likely to relapse compared with those who continued taking the medication. Most relapses occurred within the first year after cessation of treatment. Once lithium is started, it seems advisable to continue administration for at least 6 months, and preferably a year. If studies of lithium termination in adults are applicable to children, an even longer duration of treatment might be considered. Experience in adult patients with worsening of cycling and decreased response to treatment following intermittent lithium use suggests special caution regarding discontinuation of mood stabilizers. Lithium should be discontinued by gradual tapering. The clinician should closely follow up the patient after lithium is discontinued and should monitor the patient for signs of relapse so that episodes can be treated early.

Risks and Side Effects

Lithium is well tolerated by many children and adolescents, but younger children are more prone to side effects, especially at higher lithium doses and serum levels. The most common side effects in children (tremor, weight gain, headache, nausea, diarrhea) rarely require discontinuation of lithium. Polydipsia and polyuria may cause enuresis and prevent attainment of a therapeutic level. Lithium may produce goiter and/or hypothyroidism, which may have more significant consequences in developing children than in adults. Lithium effects on blood glucose level are controversial, but reactive hypoglycemia is possible. Acne may be induced or aggravated. Hypokalemia is a very rare side effect that can be managed by dietary supplementation (e.g., two bananas, two large carrots, two cups of skim milk, half of a honeydew melon, or an avocado daily), which is preferable to taking potassium tablets that taste bad and can further irritate the gastrointestinal tract. Because of its teratogenic potential, lithium is relatively contraindicated in sexually active girls.

Toxicity is closely related to serum levels, and the therapeutic margin is narrow. The patient and the family should be told to call the doctor immediately if the patient develops a febrile or gastrointestinal illness, uses rigorous dieting to lose weight, or takes diuretics or nonsteroidal anti-inflammatory agents (often taken by adolescent girls to relieve menstrual distress). Lithium should be stopped while a patient has fever, vomiting, or diarrhea. Vigorous exercise in hot weather can lead to lithium toxicity, and parents should be cautioned to make sure the patient drinks enough water. Erratic consumption of large amounts of salty snack foods may cause wide fluctuations in lithium blood levels.

■ ANTIPSYCHOTICS

Naming of this category of drugs is awkward, because many of the indications are for nonpsychotic conditions. There are two groups of these medications. The older *typical* antipsychotics, also known as *neuroleptics* or *major tranquilizers* or *first-generation antipsychotics,* include chlorpromazine (Thorazine), fluphenazine (Prolixin), haloperidol (Haldol), perphenazine (Trilafon), pimozide (Orap), thiothixene (Navane), and trifluoperazine (Stelazine). Newer medications are called *atypical* or *second generation* because they have less risk of tardive dyskinesia and other extrapyramidal side effects due to their serotonergic antagonism in addition to antidopaminergic activity. The traditional neuroleptics are primarily dopamine antagonists. The most commonly used atypicals are risperidone (Risperdal), aripiprazole (Abilify), olanzapine (Zyprexa), and quetiapine (Seroquel). Clozapine (Clozaril) is rarely used because of potentially fatal agranulocytosis and cardiomyopathy, as well as a greater risk of seizures. Ziprasidone (Geodon) carries a risk of cardiac arrhythmias, limiting its usefulness.

Indications and Efficacy

In most pediatric circumstances, an atypical would be tried first, before a typical neuroleptic, because of the side-effect profiles. However, chlorpromazine may be useful as a prn medication for agitation or acute psychosis, if sedation is needed, and thiothixene may be used if atypicals result in extreme weight gain. Risperidone, quetiapine, and aripiprazole have pediatric FDA indications for bipolar disorder, manic (age 10 years and older) and schizophrenia (13 years and older). Olanzapine has been approved for bipolar mania and schizophrenia in youth age 13 and older, with labeling that other drugs should be considered first. Risperidone and aripiprazole also have an indication for irritability in autism (ages 5–16 years and 6–17 years, respectively).

Schizophrenia

Several typical and atypical antipsychotics have modest efficacy in children and adolescents with schizophrenia. In general, however, youth with early-onset schizophrenia are less responsive to pharmacotherapy than are adults and continue to have substantial impairment, even if the positive symptoms abate. Difference in efficacy among these drugs when used for schizophrenia has not been demonstrated, with the exception of clozapine, which has been shown to benefit patients unresponsive to the other agents. Concerns about the development of tardive dyskinesia with long-term use of the typical antipsychotics and the prominence of negative symptoms in young patients with schizophrenia suggest preference for the atypicals, although they also have problematic side effects (see below). There are a number of randomized controlled trials demonstrating efficacy superior to placebo for agents in both groups of antipsychotics. Improvement in positive symptoms can be seen by the second week of treatment, but improvement in positive symptoms may not plateau for a month or longer, and negative symptoms may continue to improve for 6 months to a year.

If there is no response to a drug after a 6-week trial at adequate dose (and assured adherence), another antipsychotic (usually in a different class) may be tried. Common therapeutic errors include incorrect diagnosis, subtherapeutic or excessive medication doses, premature changes in medication, failure to monitor target symptoms or ensure adherence, hasty or irrational polypharmacy, and failure to provide psychosocial therapies in addition to medication (McClellan and Werry 1992).

Bipolar Disorder

A number of randomized controlled trials demonstrate efficacy of atypicals (aripiprazole, olanzapine, quetiapine, risperidone, and ziprasidone) as monotherapy for mania in pediatric patients with bipolar disorder. In addition, quetiapine added to valproic acid was superior to valproic acid plus placebo in adolescents with bipolar mania (DelBello et al. 2002). In a head-to-head comparison in adolescents with bipolar mania, quetiapine and valproic acid had similar efficacy, although response was faster and more patients remitted with quetiapine (DelBello et al. 2006). Monotherapy is infrequently sufficient for full remission, however, and use of more than one drug is often necessary. Compared with adults, the effect size in youth with bipolar mania is larger for the atypicals and smaller for lithium and anticonvulsant mood stabilizers.

Developmental Disorders

In doses of 0.5–4.0 mg/day, haloperidol significantly reduced hyperactivity, stereotypy, and social withdrawal in children with autism without adversely affecting cognitive performance. In addition, haloperidol improved discrimination learning and language acquisition when used in combination with positive reinforcement and behavioral interventions (Campbell et al. 1982).

Because of the more benign side-effect profile, atypicals have largely replaced typical neuroleptics. Recent multisite randomized controlled trials have shown positive results for risperidone in reducing severely disruptive behaviors in children with subaverage intelligence (Aman et al. 2002; Snyder et al. 2002). Positive effects were maintained in a 1-year open follow-up (Turgay et al. 2002). Risperidone was shown in a randomized controlled trial to reduce severe tantrums, irritability, aggression, and self-injurious behavior (but not the core symptoms of autism) in children with autistic disorder (Research Units on Pediatric Psychopharmacology Autism Network 2002).

Tourette's Disorder

Efficacy is often difficult to evaluate in Tourette's disorder because of the natural waxing and waning of symptoms. Concern about possible tardive dyskinesia from typical neuroleptics makes risperidone a more frequent choice for both aggressive symptoms and tics. If risperidone leads to excessive weight gain or is ineffective, both haloperidol and pimozide reduce tics, but discontinuation may lead to severe withdrawal exacerbation of symptoms for up to several months, and other side effects may be intolerable.

Aggressive Behavior Unresponsive to Other Interventions

Studies of hospitalized severely aggressive children ages 6–12 years have found that several typical neuroleptics are effective compared with placebo in reducing aggression, hostility, negativism, and explosiveness. The risk of cognitive dulling and tardive dyskinesia place these drugs low on the list of medication options for aggression, however. Chlorpromazine leads to unacceptable sedation at relatively low doses.

A small randomized controlled trial found low doses of risperidone to be more effective than placebo in reducing some measures of aggression in youths with conduct disorder (Findling et al. 2000).

Other Disorders

These medications, increasingly the atypicals, are used in crisis situations to decrease severe agitation, explosiveness, and aggression seen in youth with various disorders, although systematic efficacy and safety data are lacking.

Initiation and Ongoing Treatment

Before an antipsychotic medication is started, a medical history (with special focus on personal and family history of obesity, hypertension, hyperlipidemia, diabetes mellitus, and cardiovascular symptoms or disease) and a physical examination (including blood pressure, pulse, height, weight, and BMI) should be obtained. Initial laboratory studies include CBC with differential, liver functions, fasting glucose, and lipid profile. Counseling regarding nutrition and exercise should be started immediately and refreshed at every visit, if the patient's clinical condition permits. In addition to verbal discussion and opportunity for questions, published medication information sheets can be used (e.g., Dulcan 2007).

Detailed informed consent is especially crucial for clozapine and monitoring is more extensive (Towbin et al. 1994). An ECG should be obtained before starting ziprasidone, clozapine, or pimozide. An EEG is indicated before clozapine treatment because of the potential for EEG abnormalities and seizures.

The clinician should carefully examine each patient for abnormal movements with a scale such as the Abnormal Involuntary Movement Scale (AIMS) at baseline and every 3–6 months thereafter. Especially in children with autistic disorder or Tourette's disorder, it may be difficult to distinguish medication-induced movements of tardive dyskinesia or withdrawal dyskinesias from those characteristic of the disorder itself. The clinician should explain the risk of movement disorders to parents and patients (as appropriate) before starting treatment and regularly as treatment continues.

Dose must be titrated with careful attention to reduction in target symptoms and to side effects. Age, weight, and severity of symptoms do not provide clear dose guidelines. Children generally require higher mg/kg doses than adults do, and divided doses may be required in younger children. Children metabolize these drugs more rapidly, but also require lower plasma levels to be effective

(Teicher and Glod 1990). The initial dose should be very low, with gradual increments no more than once or twice a week. Loading doses or rapid titration do not accelerate clinical improvement but do increase side effects. Although a single daily dose (usually at bedtime) is generally preferred for maintenance, divided doses may be used during titration to minimize side effects and permit finer dose adjustments. Antipsychotics should be maintained at the lowest effective dose. Regular specific queries regarding side effects are required.

As treatment continues, pulse, blood pressure, height, weight, and BMI are followed at 3-month intervals. Blood triglycerides and high-density lipoprotein cholesterol (HDL) and fasting glucose are measured every 6 months. Prolactin is measured only if the patient is symptomatic (gynecomastia, galactorrhea, breast tenderness, or amenorrhea [in females]).

Risperidone, aripiprazole, and olanzapine are available as a disk (Risperdal M-Tab, Abilify Discmelt, and Zyprexa ZYDIS, respectively) that dissolves rapidly in the mouth, a useful formulation when quick drug action is needed or when pill swallowing is difficult or resisted. Risperidone, aripiprazole, and several of the typical neuroleptics are available as a liquid. Risperidone (and several typical neuroleptics) are available as a long-acting injection (Risperdal Consta). Quetiapine is available in an extended-release form (Seroquel XR).

If a typical neuroleptic is to be used, one of the higher-potency drugs, such as perphenazine or thiothixene, may be best. The lower-potency compounds (e.g., chlorpromazine) are best avoided for chronic use because of sedation, cognitive dulling, and memory deficits that can interfere with learning.

Schizophrenia

Treatment is typically started with risperidone or aripiprazole. If response is insufficient, another atypical or a typical antipsychotic is tried. Clozapine is considered only after failed treatment with two or three of the other atypicals as well as one of the typical neuroleptics. Usual starting doses for children are 0.5 mg of risperidone once or twice a day or aripiprazole 2–5 mg/day. Older adolescents with schizophrenia may require doses of antipsychotics in the adult range. Young adolescents fall in between, and doses must be individually determined. Even less is known about optimal doses of the atypical antipsychotics.

Full efficacy may not appear for up to 6 months. Positive symptoms (delusions and hallucinations) tend to decline first, followed by cognitive symptoms (thought disorder) and, very slowly, negative symptoms (apathy, anergy, withdrawal). To monitor outcome, parent and teacher reports are essential, in addition to self-reports from adolescents. Standardized clinician rating scales, such as the Positive and Negative Syndrome Scale for Schizophrenia, derived from the Children's Psychiatric Rating Scale, are sensitive to improvement in children (Spencer et al. 1994).

Current practice for adults with schizophrenia is to continue antipsychotic treatment indefinitely; however, firm recommendations regarding children are lacking because of the difficulty in making a definitive diagnosis and the possibility of developmental toxicity. Antipsychotics should be discontinued by gradual tapering to prevent rebound symptoms or relapse.

Pervasive Developmental Disorders

Unless serious side effects require immediate discontinuation, a trial of sufficient length is necessary to determine whether the drug is effective. If the drug appears to be helpful, it should be continued for at least several months. At 3- to 6-month intervals, the drug should be discontinued so that the child may be observed for withdrawal dyskinesias and to determine if the drug is still necessary.

Tourette's Disorder

Because Tourette's disorder is chronic and not usually an emergency, clinicians can carefully monitor patients for several months before starting medication. This is especially useful because of the natural waxing and waning of symptoms, and the tendency for patients to present at times of peak symptoms. A baseline of symptoms is established, and psychological and educational interventions can be implemented.

Risks and Side Effects

Pediatric patients are more prone to side effects from antipsychotic drugs than are adults, and they are at risk for prolonged exposure, including during key developmental stages. The most common and problematic side effect of the atypicals is immediate and chronic weight gain, often associated, after as short a treatment period as 12 weeks, with clinically significant hyperlipidemia and insulin resistance (Correll et al. 2009). *Metabolic syndrome,* an unfortunately common chronic complication of ongoing use of antipsychotic medication, is characterized by abdominal obesity, elevated fasting triglycerides, reduced HDL, elevated blood pressure, and elevated fasting glucose due to insulin resistance. Weight gain and associated morbidity are highest with olanzapine, quetiapine, and clozapine. Although ziprasidone causes less severe weight gain, it is associated with cortical QTc prolongation. Of the atypicals, aripiprazole has the least effect on weight.

Prolactin levels may be elevated, especially in association with risperidone and olanzapine. Sedation and cognitive dulling may exacerbate the effect of negative symptoms and interfere with school functioning. Priapism has been reported with risperidone use. Clozapine is associated with blood dyscrasias, seizures, and hypersalivation, as well as very rare myocarditis.

Acute EPS, including dystonic reactions, parkinsonian tremor and rigidity, drooling, and akathisia, are commonly seen with typical neuroleptic treatment and are more prevalent than initially hoped with atypical antipsychotic use. Laryngeal dystonia is potentially fatal. Acute dystonia may be treated with oral or intramuscular diphenhydramine (25 or 50 mg) or benztropine (0.5–2.0 mg). When medication is started in an outpatient, the clinician should instruct a responsible adult to watch for a dystonic reaction and may prescribe diphenhydramine or benztropine to use acutely if needed (or recommend an immediate visit to the local emergency room). Adolescent boys seem to be especially vulnerable to acute dystonic reactions, so prophylactic antiparkinsonian medication may be indicated (benztropine 1–2 mg/day in divided doses). Clinical experience suggests that prepubertal children do not respond well to anticholinergics, therefore reduction of antipsychotic dose is preferable to adding another drug if EPS appear. Chronic parkinsonian symptoms are often underrecognized by clinicians and may impair performance of age-appropriate activities and lead to resistance to taking medication. Although risperidone should have fewer EPS than typical neuroleptics, children appear to be more sensitive than adults to developing EPS on this drug. Very gradual dose titration may ameliorate this problem.

Akathisia may be especially difficult to identify in very young patients or those with limited verbal ability. It may be misinterpreted as anxiety or agitation and mistakenly exacerbated with an increase in antipsychotic dose. Clonazepam (Klonopin, 0.5 mg/day) may reduce neuroleptic-induced akathisia (Kutcher et al. 1987) in adolescents.

Tardive dyskinesia or withdrawal dyskinesias are frequent in children treated with typical neuroleptics (Campbell et al. 1997; Kumra et al. 1998). Most withdrawal dyskinesias are transient. Very rarely, potentially irreversible tardive dyskinesia has been documented in children and adolescents after as brief a period of treatment as 5 months. Other withdrawal-emergent symptoms include nausea, vomiting, loss of appetite, diaphoresis, and hyperactivity. Various behavioral withdrawal symptoms may appear up to several weeks after antipsychotic discontinuation and persist for as long as 8 weeks. These must be distinguished from a return of symptoms of the original disorder. Withdrawal dyskinesia has also been reported after risperidone discontinuation.

Neuroleptic malignant syndrome (NMS), a potentially fatal side effect, is manifested by hyperthermia, muscle rigidity, autonomic hyperactivity, and changes in consciousness. It has been reported to be associated with the atypicals, as well. Adolescents may present with serious medical complications or may have NMS without fever. NMS is treated by discontinuation of the antipsychotic and use of aggressive supportive measures. The use of specific medications to treat NMS has not been studied in adolescents, although case reports suggest the use of bromocriptine or dantrolene.

Abnormal laboratory findings are less often reported in children than in adults, but the clinician should be alert to the possibility of agranulocytosis or hepatic dysfunction. If an acute febrile illness or easy bruising occurs, medication should be withheld and a CBC with differential and liver enzymes should be obtained. Children may be at greater risk for drug-induced seizures than are adults, because of their immature nervous systems and the very high prevalence of abnormal EEG findings in seriously disturbed children (Teicher and Glod 1990). If excessive thirst or urination or weight loss occur, blood glucose should be measured for possible diabetes mellitus.

Of particular concern is behavioral toxicity, manifested as worsening of preexisting symptoms or development of new symptoms such as hyper- or hypoactivity, irritability, apathy, withdrawal, stereotypies, tics, or hallucinations.

Anticholinergic side effects, such as hypotension, dry mouth, constipation, nasal congestion, blurred vision, and urinary retention, are less common in children than in adults. Chlorpromazine increases the risk of sunburn.

When used for treatment of nonpsychotic disorders, haloperidol, pimozide, and risperidone have been reported to cause separation anxiety and school avoidance (Hanna et al. 1999). Side effects are a significant problem in the long-term use of haloperidol for Tourette's disorder. Frequent complaints include lethargy, feeling like a "zombie," dysphoria, personality changes, weight gain, parkinsonian symptoms, akathisia, and intellectual dulling. Some side effects of pimozide are similar to those of haloperidol but seem to be less severe. However, pimozide causes ECG changes in up to 25% of patients, including T-wave inversion, U waves, QTc prolongation, and bradycardia, although these appear to be less significant than originally thought.

■ ANTICONVULSANTS

Indications and Efficacy

Medications developed for use in the treatment of epilepsy are increasingly being used for the treatment of psychiatric symptoms, despite the lack of FDA pediatric indications. Clinical indications include bipolar disorder and severe impulsive aggression with emotional lability and irritability, with or without evidence of primary neurological findings. Although there is some supporting pediatric research, use is largely based on extrapolation from adult studies, which may not apply in younger patients. When used for these conditions, the drugs are often called *mood stabilizers,* a grouping that also includes lithium. In general, pediatric bipolar disorder seems to be less responsive to medication than in adults, and often combinations of medications are required to reduce the frequency and severity of episodes.

Sodium valproate (valproic acid [Depakene]; divalproex sodium [Depakote]) has an FDA-approved indication in adults for the treatment of mania in bipolar disorder. Evidence for effectiveness in youth includes open prospective trials, but monotherapy has not been found to be sufficiently effective for maintenance treatment (Findling et al. 2005) and an industry-sponsored randomized controlled trial failed to find divalproex extended-release to be superior to placebo in the treatment of manic or mixed episodes in youth ages 10–17 years (Wagner et al. 2009). A head-to head randomized study of quetiapine versus divalproex for adolescent mania found quetiapine to be as effective as divalproex with more rapid action (DelBello et al. 2006). A more recent randomized controlled trial found divalproex to be superior to both lithium and placebo in the treatment of youth with bipolar I disorder (Kowatch et al. 2007).

Carbamazepine (Carbatrol, Tegretol) is an older anticonvulsant that has demonstrated efficacy in adult mania, but lack of research support and problematic side effects and drug interactions limit its use in pediatric bipolar disorder. There is some evidence to support use of this drug for aggression in conduct disorder, but one controlled study did not find carbamazepine to be more effective than placebo in reducing aggression (Cueva et al. 1996). Carbamazepine has largely been replaced by the atypical antipsychotics for this use. Oxcarbazepine (Trileptal), a drug closely related to carbamazepine, has not been shown to be effective in pediatric mania (Wagner et al. 2006).

Lamotrigine (Lamictal) has an FDA indication for use in maintenance treatment to delay recurrence of manic and depressive episodes in adults with bipolar disorder. Only one published trial—an open study of lamotrigine alone or as an adjunct in adolescents with a depressive episode as part of a broad spectrum bipolar disorder—supports effectiveness in reduction of depressive symptoms (Chang et al. 2006).

Other anticonvulsants have insufficient pediatric data to recommend their use for psychiatric indications.

Initiation and Ongoing Treatment

Baseline assessments prior to using anticonvulsants, in addition to a recent pediatric history and physical examination, include menstrual and sexual history, CBC with differential and platelets, liver function tests, and a pregnancy test for postpubertal females. Of the anticonvulsants, valproate has the highest risk of teratogenicity. Prior to carbamazepine being used in patients of Asian ancestry, genetic testing is recommended for HLA-B*1502, an allele that increases risk of dangerous skin reactions.

Valproate

For children and adolescents, valproate is typically started at 10–15 mg/kg/day in two or three divided doses and then titrated up gradually according to tolerance and response. Serum valproate levels are optimally measured 12 hours after the last dose. Target serum levels for treating mania are thought to be 80–110 μg/mL. Depakote is often the preferred formulation (over Depakene) because it is enteric-coated to reduce gastrointestinal side effects. An extended-release formulation (Depakote ER) permits fewer daily doses. A soft-gel capsule of valproic acid delayed release (Stavzor) is easier to swallow.

Coadministration of guanfacine has been shown to increase plasma levels of valproate (Ambrosini and Sheikh 1998). This is more relevant now that an extended-release form of guanfacine (Intuniv) has been approved with an indication for ADHD.

Carbamazepine

Typical starting dose is 15 mg/kg/day or for children 100 mg twice a day and for adolescents 100 mg three times a day. Dose may be increased by 100–200 mg/day at weekly intervals. The maximum total daily dose of carbamazepine is 1,000 mg in children and 1,200 mg in adolescents. Usual maintenance doses are 10–20 mg/kg/day divided into two or three doses per day. There is an extended release form (Equetro) that permits one dose per day. There are no systematic data on optimal therapeutic levels for treatment of pediatric aggression or bipolar disorder. The commonly used maintenance level is 7–10 µg/mL.

Risks and Side Effects

Data on pediatric safety and tolerability of the anticonvulsants are mostly derived from experience with the use of these drugs in the treatment of epilepsy. Behavioral toxicity is possible with any of these drugs (more likely with carbamazepine and gabapentin). Lamotrigine is associated with Stevens-Johnson syndrome, a potentially fatal allergic skin reaction. The risk is increased when lamotrigine is combined with valproate. In 2010, the FDA mandated a warning regarding association of lamotrigine with aseptic meningitis. Phenobarbital is associated with impaired memory and attention, learning disorders, hyperactivity, irritability, aggression, and depressed mood. Topiramate may cause cognitive dulling and memory problems. Drug interactions between anticonvulsants and other medications are often problematic.

The FDA has placed a warning on all anticonvulsants of increased risk of suicidal thoughts and behavior.

Valproate

Common side effects include gastrointestinal symptoms, weight gain, sedation, transient hair loss, and tremor. Rare and serious adverse effects include liver toxicity (primarily in children younger than 3 years who are taking multiple anticonvulsants, usually reversible when the drug is stopped), hyperammonemia, blood dyscrasias, and very rare pancreatitis. Patients should be monitored for nausea, vomiting, easy bruising, lethargy, disorientation, malaise, or persistent abdominal pain (possible pancreatitis). Significant concern has been raised by the connection between valproate use and polycystic ovary syndrome, manifested by obesity, insulin resistance, acne, hirsutism, and irregular or absent menstrual periods (associated with decreased fertility), and female patients should be monitored closely for these symptoms.

Valproate is contraindicated in pregnancy because of increased rates of developmental delay and neural tube defects in exposed babies. The drug should not be used in sexually active females in the absence of highly reliable use of birth control.

Carbamazepine

Common side effects include nausea, vomiting, vertigo, decreased coordination, drowsiness, blurred vision, and nystagmus (reversible by lowering dose). Rare adverse events include tics, ataxia, blood dyscrasias, decreased thyroid function, hepatitis, exacerbation of seizures, and life-threatening skin reaction. Adverse behavioral reactions may occur, with mania, extreme irritability, agitation, insomnia, obsessive thinking, hallucinations, delirium, psychosis, paranoia, hyperactivity, and aggression, especially in the first month of treatment. Carbamazepine is contraindicated in pregnancy or risk of pregnancy because of teratogenicity.

■ MELATONIN

Melatonin is a naturally occurring neurotransmitter related to serotonin and tryptophan. It influences circadian rhythms in the anterior hypothalamus and is capable of shifting sleep phase. Melatonin is frequently recommended by physicians or used independently by parents for initial insomnia (delayed sleep onset) in typically developing children and in youth with initial insomnia comorbid with ADHD, autism spectrum disorders, and neurodevelopmental disabilities, as well as in adolescents with delayed sleep phase syndrome. In a randomized controlled trial in children ages 6–12 years with chronic (1 year or more) sleep-onset insomnia, 5 mg of melatonin given at 7 P.M. was superior to placebo, on average decreasing sleep latency by 17 minutes and advancing sleep onset by 57 minutes (Smits et al. 2003). Total sleep time did not change. Health status improvement in the melatonin condition was greater than with placebo. A substantial proportion of the subjects had ADHD, some taking methylphenidate and some unmedicated for ADHD. In a study of children (6–14 years old, 91% boys) with ADHD and initial insomnia (Weiss et al. 2006), all being treated with stimulants, the first intervention was sleep hygiene modifications for all. Those with insufficient response (continued mean or intermittent sleep latency of more than 60 minutes) (23 of 28 subjects) entered a double-blind crossover trial of placebo versus 5 mg pharmaceutical-grade melatonin given 20 minutes before bedtime. Relative to placebo, melatonin decreased initial insomnia by 16 minutes. Combined sleep hygiene and melatonin resulted in a mean decrease in initial insomnia of 60 minutes. Adverse events did not differ from placebo. Interestingly, improved sleep did not show an effect on ADHD symptoms.

In the treatment of initial insomnia, melatonin is given approximately 30 minutes before desired sleep-onset time. One may start with a dose of 1.5 mg and increase in 1.5-mg increments every 4–5 days as needed, to a dose of 10–15 mg. Lower doses are used to normalize the circadian sleep-wake cycle in delayed sleep phase syndrome. Approximately 0.3 mg is given about 4–5 hours before the current habitual time of falling asleep. The same dose is gradually moved earlier as the falling asleep time is moved earlier (advanced).

Melatonin is not regulated as a drug and is sold as a food or nutritional supplement over the counter, raising concerns about variable potency of preparations and possible impurities. Side effects of melatonin per se are minimal, if any.

■ REFERENCES

Alessi N, Naylor MW, Ghaziuddin M, et al: Update on lithium carbonate therapy in children and adolescents. J Am Acad Child Adolesc Psychiatry 33:291–304, 1994

Allen AJ, Kurlan RM, Gilbert DL, et al: Atomoxetine treatment in children and adolescents with ADHD and comorbid tic disorders. Neurology 65:1941–1949, 2006

Aman MG, Smedt GD, Derivan A, et al: Double-blind, placebo-controlled study of risperidone for the treatment of disruptive behaviors in children with subaverage intelligence. Am J Psychiatry 159:1337–1346, 2002

Ambrosini PJ, Sheikh RM: Increased plasma valproate concentrations when coadministered with guanfacine. J Child Adolesc Psychopharmacol 8:143–147, 1998

Barrickman LL, Perry PH, Allen AJ, et al: Bupropion versus methylphenidate in the treatment of attention-deficit hyperactivity disorder. J Am Acad Child Adolesc Psychiatry 34:649–657, 1995

Biederman J, Melmed RD, Patel A, et al: A randomized, double-blind, placebo-controlled study of guanfacine extended release in children and adolescents with attention-deficit/hyperactivity disorder. Pediatrics 121:e73–e84, 2008

Birmaher B, Axelson DA, Monk K, et al: Fluoxetine for the treatment of childhood anxiety disorders. J Am Acad Child Adolesc Psychiatry 42:415–423, 2003

Black B, Uhde TW: Treatment of elective mutism with fluoxetine: a double-blind, placebo-controlled study. J Am Acad Child Adolesc Psychiatry 33:1000–1006, 1994

Bloch MH, Panza KE, Landeros-Weisenberger A, et al: Meta-analysis: treatment of attention-deficit/hyperactivity disorder in children with comorbid tic disorders. J Am Acad Child Adolesc Psychiatry 48:884–893, 2009

Brent D, Emslie G, Wagner KD, et al: Switching to another SSRI or to venlafaxine with or without cognitive behavioral therapy for adolescents with SSRI-resistant depression: The TORDIA Randomized Controlled Trial. JAMA 299:901–913, 2008

Campbell M, Anderson LT, Small AM, et al: The effects of haloperidol on learning and behavior in autistic children. J Autism Dev Disord 12:167–175, 1982

Campbell M, Armenteros JL, Malone RP, et al: Neuroleptic-related dyskinesias in autistic children: a prospective, longitudinal study. J Am Acad Child Adolesc Psychiatry 36:835–843, 1997

Chang K, Saxena K, Howe M: An open-label study of lamotrigine adjunct or monotherapy for the treatment of adolescents with bipolar depression. J Am Acad Child Adolesc Psychiatry 45:298–304, 2006

Connor DF, Barkley RA, Davis HT: A pilot study of methylphenidate, clonidine, or the combination in ADHD comorbid with aggressive oppositional defiant or conduct disorder. Clin Pediatr 39:15–25, 2000

Correll CU, Manu P, Olshanskiy V, et al: Cardiometabolic risk of second-generation antipsychotic medications during first-time use in children and adolescents. JAMA 302:1765–1773, 2009

Cueva JE, Overall JE, Small AM, et al: Carbamazepine in aggressive children with conduct disorder: a double-blind and placebo-controlled study. J Am Acad Child Adolesc Psychiatry 35:480–490, 1996

DelBello MP, Schwiers L, Rosenberg HL, et al: A double-blind, randomized, placebo-controlled study of quetiapine as adjunctive treatment for adolescent mania. J Am Acad Child Adolesc Psychiatry 41:1216–1223, 2002

DelBello MP, Kowatch RA, Adler CM, et al: A double-blind randomized pilot study comparing quetiapine and divalproex for adolescent mania. J Am Acad Child Adolesc Psychiatry 45:305–313, 2006

Donnelly M, Rapoport JL: Attention deficit disorders, in Diagnosis and Psychopharmacology of Childhood and Adolescent Disorders. Edited by Weiner JM. New York, Wiley, 1985, pp 178–197

Dulcan MK (ed): Helping Parents, Youth, and Teachers Understand Medications for Behavioral and Emotional Problems: A Resource Book of Medication Information Handouts, 3rd Edition. Washington, DC, American Psychiatric Publishing, 2007

Efron D, Jarman F, Barker M: Side effects of methylphenidate and dextroamphetamine in children with attention deficit hyperactivity disorder: a double-blind, crossover trial. Pediatrics 100:662–666, 1997

Elia J, Borcherding BG, Rapoport JL, et al: Methylphenidate and dextroamphetamine treatment of hyperactivity: are there true nonresponders? Psychiatry Res 36:141–155, 1991

Faraone SV, Biederman J, Morley CP, et al: Effect of stimulants on height and weight: a review of the literature. J Am Acad Child Adolesc Psychiatry 47:994–1009, 2008

Findling RL, McNamara NK, Branicky LA, et al: A double-blind pilot study of risperidone in the treatment of conduct disorder. J Am Acad Child Adolesc Psychiatry 39:509–516, 2000

Findling RL, McNamara NK, Youngstrom EA, et al: Double-blind 18-month trial of lithium versus divalproex maintenance treatment in pediatric bipolar disorder. J Am Acad Child Adolesc Psychiatry 44:409–417, 2005

Geller B, Fetner HH: Children's 24-hour serum lithium level after a single dose predicts initial dose and steady state plasma levels. J Clin Psychopharmacol 9:155, 1989

Greenhill L, Kollins, S, Abikoff H, et al: Efficacy and safety of immediate-release methylphenidate treatment for preschoolers with ADHD. J Am Acad Child Adolesc Psychiatry 45:1284–1293, 2006

Hanna GL, Fluent TE, Fischer DJ: Case report: separation anxiety in children and adolescents treated with risperidone. J Child Adolesc Psychopharmacol 9:277–283, 1999

Hollander E, Phillips A, Chaplin W, et al: A placebo controlled crossover trial of liquid fluoxetine on repetitive behaviors in childhood and adolescent autism. Neuropsychopharmacology 30:582–589, 2005

Hughes CW, Emslie GJ, Crismon ML, et al: Texas Children's Medication Algorithm Project: update from Texas Consensus Conference Panel on Medication Treatment of Childhood Major Depressive Disorder. J Am Acad Child Adolesc Psychiatry 46:667–686, 2007

Hunt RD: Treatment effects of oral and transdermal clonidine in relation to methylphenidate—an open pilot study in ADHD. Psychopharmacol Bull 23:111–114, 1987

Jain R, Segal S, Kollins SH, et al: Clonidine extended-release tablets for pediatric patients with attention-deficit/hyperactivity disorder. J Am Acad Child Adolesc Psychiatry 50:171–179, 2011

Kelsey DK, Sumner CR, Casat CD, et al: Once-daily atomoxetine treatment of children with ADHD, including an assessment of evening and morning behavior: a double-blind, placebo-controlled trial. Pediatrics 114:e1–e8, 2004

Kent JD, Blader JC, Koplewicz HS, et al: Effects of late-afternoon methylphenidate administration on behavior and sleep in attention-deficit hyperactivity disorder. Pediatrics 96:320–325, 1995

King BH, Hollander E, Sikich L: Lack of efficacy of citalopram in children with autism spectrum disorders and high levels of repetitive behavior: citalopram ineffective in children with autism. Arch Gen Psychiatry 66:583–590, 2009

Kowatch R, Findling R, Scheffer R, et al: Placebo controlled trial of divalproex versus lithium for bipolar disorder. Presented at the annual meeting of the American Academy of Child and Adolescent Psychiatry, Boston, MA, October 2007

Kumra S, Jacobsen LK, Lenane M, et al: Case series: spectrum of neuroleptic-induced movement disorders and extrapyramidal side effects in childhood-onset schizophrenia. J Am Acad Child Adolesc Psychiatry 37:221–227, 1998

Kurlan R: Methylphenidate to treat ADHD is not contraindicated in children with tics. Mov Disord 17:5–6, 2002

Kutcher SP, MacKenzie S, Galarraga W, et al: Clonazepam treatment of adolescents with neuroleptic-induced akathisia. Am J Psychiatry 144:823–824, 1987

Lake MB, Birmaher B, Wassick S, et al: Case report: bleeding and selective serotonin reuptake inhibitors in childhood and adolescence. J Child Adolesc Psychopharmacol 10:35–38, 2000

March JS, Entusah AR, Rynn M, et al: A randomized controlled trial of venlafaxine ER versus placebo in pediatric social anxiety disorder. Biol Psychiatry 62:1149–1154, 2007

McClellan JM, Werry JS: Schizophrenia. Psychiatr Clin North Am 15:131–148, 1992

Meighen KG: Duloxetine treatment of pediatric chronic pain and co-morbid major depressive disorder. J Child Adolesc Psychopharmacol 17:121–127, 2007

Michelson D, Faries D, Wernicke J, et al: Atomoxetine in the treatment of children and adolescents with attention-deficit/hyperactivity disorder: a randomized, placebo-controlled, dose-response study. Pediatrics 108:e83, 2001

Mrakotsky C, Masek B, Biederman J, et al: Prospective open-label pilot trial of mirtazapine in children and adolescents with social phobia. J Anxiety Disord 22:88–97, 2008

MTA Cooperative Group: 14-month randomized clinical trial of treatment strategies for attention- deficit/hyperactivity disorder. Arch Gen Psychiatry 56:1073–1086, 1999

Newcorn JH, Spencer TJ, Biederman J, et al: Atomoxetine treatment in children and adolescents with attention-deficit/hyperactivity disorder and comorbid oppositional defiant disorder. J Am Acad Child Adolesc Psychiatry 44:240–248, 2005

Newcorn JH, Sutton VK, Weiss MD, et al: Clinical responses to atomoxetine in attention-deficit/hyperactivity disorder: the Integrated Data Exploratory Analysis (IDEA) Study. J Am Acad Child Adolesc Psychiatry 48:511–518, 2009

Palumbo DR, Sallee FR, Pelham WE, et al: Clonidine for attention-deficit/hyperactivity disorder, I: efficacy and tolerability outcomes. J Am Acad Child Adolesc Psychiatry 47:180–188, 2008

Perrin JM, Friedman R, Knilans TK, et al: Cardiovascular monitoring and stimulant drugs for attention-deficit/hyperactivity disorder. Pediatrics 122:451–453, 2008

Pliszka SR, Greenhill LL, Crismon ML, et al: The Texas Children's Medication Algorithm Project: report of the Texas Consensus Conference Panel on Medication Treatment of Childhood Attention-Deficit/Hyperactivity Disorder, Part II: tactics. J Am Acad Child Adolesc Psychiatry 39:920–927, 2000

Research Units on Pediatric Psychopharmacology Autism Network: Risperidone in children with autism and serious behavioral problems. N Engl J Med 347:314–321, 2002

Rynn MA, Siqueland L, Rickels K: Placebo-controlled trial of sertraline in the treatment of children with generalized anxiety disorder. Am J Psychiatry 158:2008–2014, 2001

Sallee FR, McGough J, Wigal T, et al: Guanfacine extended release in children and adolescents with attention-deficit/hyperactivity disorder: a placebo-controlled trial. J Am Acad Child Adolesc Psychiatry 48:155–165, 2009

Scahill L, Chappell PB, Kim YS, et al: A placebo-controlled study of guanfacine in the treatment of children with tic disorders and attention deficit hyperactivity disorder. Am J Psychiatry 158:1067–1074, 2001

Smits MG, van Stel HF, van der Heijden K, et al: Melatonin improves health status and sleep in children with idiopathic chronic sleep-onset insomnia: a randomized placebo-controlled trial. J Am Acad Child Adolesc Psychiatry 42:1286–1293, 2003

Snyder R, Turgay A, Aman M, et al: Effects of risperidone on conduct and disruptive behavior disorders in children with subaverage IQs. J Am Acad Child Adolesc Psychiatry 41:1026–1036, 2002

Spencer EK, Alpert M, Pouget ER: Scales for the assessment of neuroleptic response in schizophrenic children: specific measures derived from the CPRS. Psychopharmacol Bull 30:199–202, 1994

Strober M, Morrell W, Lampert C, et al: A family study of bipolar I illness in adolescence: early onset of symptoms linked to increased familial loading and lithium resistance. J Affect Disord 15:255–268, 1988

Strober M, Morrell W, Lampert C, et al: Relapse following discontinuation of lithium maintenance therapy in adolescents with bipolar I illness: a naturalistic study. Am J Psychiatry 147:457–461, 1990

Teicher MH, Glod CA: Neuroleptic drugs: indications and guidelines for their rational use in children and adolescents. J Child Adolesc Psychopharmacol 1:33–56, 1990

Tourette's Syndrome Study Group: Treatment of ADHD in children with tics: a randomized controlled trial. Neurology 58:527–536, 2002

Towbin KE, Dykens EM, Pugliese RG: Clozapine for early developmental delays with childhood-onset schizophrenia: protocol and 15-month outcome. J Am Acad Child Adolesc Psychiatry 33:651–657, 1994

Turgay A, Binder C, Snyder R, et al: Long-term safety and efficacy of risperidone for the treatment of disruptive behavior disorders in children with subaverage IQs. Pediatrics 110:1–12, 2002

Vitiello B: Developmental aspects of pediatric psychopharmacology, in Clinical Manual of Child and Adolescent Psychopharmacology. Edited by Findling RL. Washington, DC, American Psychiatric Publishing, 2008, pp 1–31

Wagner KD, Berard R, Stein MB, et al: A multicenter, randomized, double-blind, placebo-controlled trial of paroxetine in children and adolescents with social anxiety disorder. Arch Gen Psychiatry 61:1153–1162, 2004

Wagner KD, Kowatch RA, Emslie GJ, et al: A double-blind, randomized, placebo-controlled trial of oxcarbazepine in the treatment of bipolar disorder in children and adolescents. Am J Psychiatry 163:1179–1186, 2006

Wagner KD, Redden L, Kowatch RA, et al: A double-blind, randomized, placebo-controlled trial of divalproex extended-release in the treatment of bipolar disorder in children and adolescents. J Am Acad Child Adolesc Psychiatry 48:519–532, 2009

Walkup JT, Labellarte MJ, Riddle MA, et al: Fluvoxamine for the treatment of anxiety disorders in children and adolescents. N Engl J Med 344:1279–1285, 2001

Walkup JT, Albano AM, Piacentini J, et al: Cognitive behavioral therapy, sertraline, or a combination in childhood anxiety. N Engl J Med 359:2753–2766, 2008

Weiss MD, Wasdell MB, Bomben MM, et al: Sleep hygiene and melatonin treatment for children and adolescents with ADHD and initial insomnia. J Am Acad Child Adolesc Psychiatry 45:512–519, 2006

Weller EB, Weller RA, Fristad MA: Lithium dosage guide for prepubertal children: a preliminary report. J Am Acad Child Adolesc Psychiatry 25:92–95, 1986

Wilens TE, Spencer TJ: Combining methylphenidate and clonidine: a clinically sound medication option. J Am Acad Child Adolesc Psychiatry 38:614–616, 1999

Wilens TE, Bukstein O, Cutler AJ, et al: A multicenter placebo-controlled study of extended-release guanfacine coadministered with psychostimulants in the treatment of attention-deficit/hyperactivity disorder: effects on overall, morning, and evening ADHD assessments. Poster presented at the annual meeting of the American Academy of Child and Adolescent Psychiatry, New York City, October 2010

■ ADDITIONAL READING

American Academy of Child and Adolescent Psychiatry: Practice parameter for the assessment and treatment of children and adolescents with attention-deficit/hyperactivity disorder. J Am Acad Child Adolesc Psychiatry 46:894–921, 2007

American Academy of Child and Adolescent Psychiatry: Practice parameter on the use of psychotropic medication in children and adolescents. J Am Acad Child Adolesc Psychiatry 48:961–973, 2009

Dulcan MK (ed): Part X: Somatic Treatments, in Dulcan's Textbook of Child and Adolescent Psychiatry. Washington, DC, American Psychiatric Publishing, 2010, pp 667–794

Findling RL (ed): Clinical Manual of Child and Adolescent Psychopharmacology. Washington, DC, American Psychiatric Publishing, 2008

9

PSYCHOSOCIAL TREATMENTS

The ideal mental health service delivery system provides a continuum of care (i.e., integrated programs at all levels of intensity). The child and family can move easily from one service to another as the clinical situation warrants.

Child and adolescent psychiatric disorders cannot be successfully treated unless the family dynamics and the school environment are considered. The parents are always involved, at a minimum to ensure coordinated treatment and to remove any secondary gain caused by the child's symptoms. For many disorders, therapeutic work with the parents or the family is just as important, or even more important, than direct therapy with the child. Often, the therapist coordinates with the school, the pediatrician, a social welfare agency, juvenile court personnel, and/or a community recreation leader. Whatever the modalities of therapy used, the therapist must be aware of the patient's level of physical, cognitive, and emotional development in order to understand the symptoms, set appropriate goals, and tailor effective interventions. A focus on the skills necessary for successful development and adaptation, with attention to improving those at which the child and parent are not sufficiently competent, may facilitate successful therapy (see Strayhorn 1988 in "Additional Reading").

In the outpatient setting, treatment by a single therapist is generally most efficient and effective. Indications for collaborative treatment (two or more therapists working as a team) include an adolescent who is unusually concerned about confidentiality, the need for different types of skills that one therapist does not have, or a clear need of the patient and parent(s) for different qualities in a therapist (e.g., the child would benefit from a male role model, but the mother has great difficulty relating to men). In collaborative treatment, the therapists must maintain free and open communication, discuss and agree on treatment plans, and avoid aligning into competitive "teams." Unresolved conflicts over relative power and authority of the therapists will lead to difficulties in treatment.

Therapists must maintain clear guidelines for confidentiality and for relaying information between the parent and child. Adolescents are usually more sensitive to this issue than children. In general, the therapist should tell either party when and what information from his or her session will be relayed to the other. In some situations, parents and children may participate in the decision or in the communication itself. When children or adolescents are engaging in potentially dangerous activities or have serious thoughts of harming themselves or others, parents must be informed. Carefully planned joint parent–child sessions, in which the therapist coaches and supports the parent or child in sharing information, may be more useful than reports from the therapist.

Recommended books and chapters in "Additional Reading" offer guidance in implementing treatments.

■ COMMUNICATION WITH CHILDREN AND ADOLESCENTS

Children's ability to use language is limited by their cognitive immaturity. Young children often use play to express feelings, to narrate past events, and to work through trauma. In play therapy, the therapist uses the metaphor of the child's symbolic play and bases questions and comments on characters in the play rather than focusing directly on the child's own feelings and experiences (even if the connection is clear to the therapist). The skilled therapist tailors communication to the child's stage of language and cognitive development and must be aware that the vocabulary of some bright and precocious children exceeds their emotional understanding of events and concepts. Dramatic play with dolls or puppets; drawing and other art techniques; and questions about dreams, wishes, or favorite stories or television shows can provide access to children's fantasies, emotions, and concerns.

■ THE RESISTANT CHILD OR ADOLESCENT

It is not surprising that many children and adolescents do not cooperate in therapy. Most are brought to treatment by adults and often do not perceive a reason for change; they view it as "giving in" to parents or teachers. In addition, a child or an adolescent may refuse to participate in or attempt to sabotage therapy for various dynamic reasons. Strategies to reduce resistance are more effective if tailored to the cause. A child who is anxious or having difficulty separating from a parent may be helped by having the parent initially present in therapy. The therapist may address, either directly or through play, the patient's reluctance to participate and may suggest possible causes that the child is unwilling or unable to verbalize. Long silences are generally not helpful and tend to lead to increased anxiety or struggle for control. Attractive play materials help to make the therapy situation less threatening and to encourage participation while the therapist builds an alliance. Even adolescents often appreciate the availability of paper and markers. Play can be combined with therapy in techniques such as storytelling, drama, and specially designed games. The therapist must guard, however, against the danger of the sessions becoming mere play or recreation instead of therapy. Use of a token economy in the therapy situation may improve motivation, especially for materially deprived or oppositional children.

■ TYPES OF PSYCHOTHERAPY

The common themes of individual therapies are listed in Table 9–1.

Supportive Therapy

Supportive therapy may be especially useful for children and adolescents who do not have satisfying relationships with adults be-

TABLE 9–1.	**Common themes of individual therapies**

A relationship with a therapist who is identified as a helping person and who has some degree of control and influence over the patient

Instillation of hope, pride, and improved morale

Use of attention, encouragement, and suggestion

Goals of helping the patient to achieve greater control, competence, mastery, autonomy, and coping skills

Goals to abandon or modify unrealistic expectations of self, others, and the environment

Source. Adapted from Strupp 1973.

cause their symptoms make it very difficult to establish a positive relationship or their parents are emotionally or physically unavailable, or even hostile. For the patient in crisis, the therapist provides support until a stressor resolves, a developmental crisis has passed, or the patient or environment changes sufficiently that other adults can take on the supportive role. The patient has a real relationship with the therapist, who facilitates catharsis and provides understanding and judicious advice.

Psychodynamically Oriented Therapy

Psychodynamically oriented therapy is grounded in psychoanalytic theory but is more flexible and emphasizes the real relationship with the therapist, the provision of a corrective emotional experience, and the experience of transference. Goals include resolution of symptoms, change in behavior, and resumption of the normal developmental process. Mechanisms of change include understanding and working with transference feelings, catharsis, development of insight, strengthening of ego skills and adaptive defenses, and improvement in reality testing. The therapist forms an alliance with the child or adolescent, identifies feelings, clarifies thoughts and events, makes interpretations, judiciously gives information and advice, and acts as an advocate for the patient. Sessions are held once or twice a week.

Possible candidates for psychodynamically oriented individual therapy include verbal youngsters (or those who can use symbolic play) who are in significant emotional distress or who are struggling to deal with a stressor or traumatic event (e.g., parental death, divorce, or abandonment; physical illness). Patients with attention-deficit/hyperactivity disorder (ADHD) or disruptive behavior disorders are unlikely to benefit. Youngsters with ADHD have little insight into their behavior and its effect on others and may be genuinely unable to report their problems or to reflect on them. Patients with oppositional defiant and conduct disorders refuse to acknowledge problem behavior and are better treated in family or group therapy or in a structured milieu.

Time-Limited Therapy

All the models of time-limited therapy have in common a planned relatively brief duration (several sessions to 6 months), a predominant focus on the present, and a high degree of structure and attention to specific, limited goals. Theoretical foundations of various models include psychodynamic, crisis, family systems, cognitive, behavioral or social learning, and guidance or educational. Both the therapist and the patient must take active roles. The short duration is used to increase patient motivation and participation and limit nonadaptive dependency and regression. A great deal of attention is paid to the process of termination and to how the patient will continue to make progress after therapy stops. Psychodynamic models emphasize a firm termination of therapy, while cognitive, behavioral, and supportive models often include periodic "booster" sessions.

Time-limited treatment appears to be at least as effective as longer-term therapy for some patients. Time-limited methods have been recommended for multiproblem, crisis-oriented families who are unlikely to persist in longer-term treatment and for well-functioning children and families with circumscribed problems of recent onset. Brief treatment is relatively contraindicated for long-standing severe problems and for children and adolescents who have endured serious losses and/or deprivation.

Other Models of Therapy

Specific structured therapy programs and techniques have been developed and tested for a variety of pediatric psychiatric disorders and symptoms (see "Additional Reading"). These techniques may be used individually or in diagnosis-specific groups. Parents may be included in psychoeducation, support, implementation of strategies at home, and/or interventions for their own symptoms, to improve outcome for the youth.

Cognitive-Behavioral Therapy

Manualized cognitive-behavioral therapy (CBT) techniques have been developed and adapted for children and adolescents with many disorders, including depression, obsessive-compulsive disorder, posttraumatic stress disorder, anxiety disorders, and bulimia nervosa. These techniques may be used individually, in diagnosis-specific group therapy settings, or in family based treatment (see Chorpita 2007 in "Additional Reading").

CBT encompasses a range of techniques used to target specific symptoms. The key components include exposure and response prevention (a hierarchy of feared situations is gradually and successfully approached with graduated exposures), cognitive restructuring (recognition of negative thought processes that are then challenged and replaced with more realistic and positive self-statements to improve emotional/behavioral responses to situations), relaxation training (reducing arousal by progressive use of relaxation exercises or cognitive meditation techniques), pleasant activity scheduling or behavioral activation (particularly for patients with anergia, anhedonia, lack of motivation, or social isolation), and problem-solving skills (exercises to sequentially examine problems, goals, and possible solutions, with selection of an agreed-upon strategy to employ and subsequent self-evaluation of the results). Parents and caregivers can play a critical "coaching" role for CBT assignments between sessions and their collaboration is essential in psychoeducation and treatment planning.

Interpersonal Psychotherapy

Interpersonal psychotherapy for depressed adolescents (IPT-A) was developed as a time-limited psychotherapy based on the work of interpersonal theorists and developmental adaptation from the interpersonal psychotherapy (IPT) as used with adults. The IPT model focuses on the premise that depression occurs within an interpersonal framework. IPT serves to relieve symptoms of depression by improving communication patterns, which then positively influence relationships, thus improving depression. IPT also incorporates attachment theory by addressing interpersonal conflicts, transitions, and grief in the context of relationships. IPT-A was designed as a 12-week treatment for nonpsychotic depressed adolescents. It has been used when comorbidities exist, although it is most effective when depression is the primary diagnosis and comorbidities are minimal (Gunlicks-Stoessel and Mufson 2010). Parental participation is recommended (see Mufson et al. 2004 in "Additional Reading").

Motivational Interviewing

Motivational interviewing has its roots in the work of Carl Rogers on client-centered therapy. It is particularly useful with patients who do not come to treatment of their own accord, such as adolescents who abuse substances. The basic principle is that if a person experiences a safe, comfortable, and collaborative therapeutic environment, he or she will be more likely to participate with the therapist to acknowledge and examine his or her problems and make progress toward their resolution. Techniques deal explicitly with patient resistance and ambivalence to enhance motivation and willingness to consider change in behavior (see Nagy 2010 in "Additional Reading").

Dialectical Behavior Therapy

Dialectical behavior therapy (DBT), based on the theoretical and empirical work of Linehan with adults suffering from borderline

320

personality disorder, has been developmentally extended to work with suicidal adolescents (see Miller et al. 2007 in "Additional Reading"). This approach combines creative individual, family, and group interventions from a variety of conceptual frameworks in the treatment of this very difficult and crisis-prone population.

■ PARENT COUNSELING AND PSYCHOEDUCATION

Parent counseling or guidance is primarily an educational intervention, conducted with individual parents or couples in groups. Parents learn about normal child development. The therapist helps parents to understand their child and his or her problems and to modify parental attitudes and behaviors that seem to be contributing to the difficulties. The therapist must try to understand the parents' point of view and to be sympathetic to the hardships of living with a disturbed child or adolescent. For parents who have serious difficulties of their own, parent counseling may merge into or pave the way for marital therapy or individual treatment of the adult.

Virtually all parents of children with psychiatric or learning problems need and deserve education on the nature of their child's disorder and how to select among treatments and manage difficult behavior. Parents spend far more time with their children than the therapist does and can powerfully assist or impede treatment. Parents of children with chronic problems must become skilled advocates, to ensure that their children receive the treatment and schooling that they need. Carefully selected reading material ("bibliotherapy") may be extremely useful to parents (see Appendix).

■ BEHAVIOR THERAPY

Behavioral therapists view symptoms as resulting from habits, faulty learning, inappropriate environmental responses to behavior, or neurodevelopmental deficits, rather than from unconscious or intrapsychic motivation. Behavior therapy is characterized by detailed assessment of problematic behaviors and the environmental conditions that elicit and maintain them, the development of strategies to produce change in the environment and therefore in the patient's behavior, and repeated assessment to evaluate the success of the intervention.

In an operant approach, positive and negative environmental contingencies (responses to the child's behavior) are identified and then modified in an attempt to decrease problem behaviors and increase adaptive ones. A *token economy* is one type of operant approach, in which points, stickers, or tokens can be earned for desirable behaviors (and lost for problem behaviors) and then exchanged for backup reinforcers (e.g., money, food, toys, privileges, or time with an adult in a pleasant activity). Token economies can be used successfully by parents, teachers, therapists (with groups or individuals), and staff of inpatient or day treatment programs.

Social learning theory integrates operant conditioning theory with an understanding of cognitive processes and emphasizes the importance of learning new behaviors by observing or imitating others. For example, modeling is used in the treatment of children's anxiety and fears to decrease social withdrawal and teach adaptive skills.

Indications and Efficacy

Behavior therapy is by far the most thoroughly evaluated psychological treatment for children. It is the most effective treatment for simple phobias (using systematic desensitization), for enuresis and encopresis, and for a wide range of noncompliant behaviors. Maximally effective programs require home and school cooperation, focus on specific target behaviors, and implement contingencies quickly and consistently following behavior. Potential problems in the use of behavior therapy are the lack of maintenance of improvement over time and the failure to generalize the new behaviors to situations other than the ones in which training occurred. Generalization can be maximized by conducting training at varied times and places in the settings in which behavior change is desired, facilitating transfer to naturally occurring reinforcers, developing new reinforcers in the child's environment, and gradually fading reinforcement on an intermittent schedule.

Parent Management Training

Empirically tested effective training packages are available to teach parents to use behavior modification techniques to manage noncompliant, oppositional, and aggressive children (for example, see Forehand and McMahon 2003 and Webster-Stratton and Herbert 1994 in "Additional Reading"). Parents are taught to give clear instructions, to positively reinforce good behavior, and to use punishment effectively. Teaching techniques include written and verbal instruction in social learning principles and the use of behavior modification programs; modeling by the therapist; behavioral rehearsal of skills to be used; and homework assignments with subsequent review, feedback, and repetition. One frequently used negative contingency is the time-out, so called because it puts the child in a quiet, boring area where he or she experiences a "time-out" from accidental or naturally occurring positive reinforcement.

Treatment is most effective for young children and those with less severe and persistent behavior problems. Characteristics that have been associated with less positive outcome in parent training include low socioeconomic status, parental psychiatric problems, marital conflict, lack of a social support network, harsh punishment practices, and parent history of antisocial behavior (Kazdin 1997). Families with these characteristics should receive maximally potent interventions, with attention to the parents' individual or marital problems as necessary. Additional topics may need to be addressed, such as skills for resolving marital conflict or managing parental anger. More highly functioning families may be able to succeed with written materials only or by using manuals or videotapes supplemented by group discussion. The therapist must be aware of ethnic and cultural beliefs and customs regarding child development and parenting.

Behavioral intervention can be done in the context of family therapy, including techniques such as parent–child contingency contracting. A social contract is written that specifies the behaviors that the parent and child will change, with contingencies. The family is trained to negotiate and problem-solve. These techniques may be particularly useful for adolescents.

Classroom Behavior Modification

Techniques for use in schools include class rules, attention to positive behavior, token economies, and response-cost programs (reinforcers are withdrawn in response to undesirable behavior). One successful program for children with attention and conduct problems required only that the teacher observe the child for off-task behavior and give verbal feedback every 30 minutes (Pelham and Murphy 1986). The teacher may dispense simple reinforcers such as praise, stars on a chart, or classroom privileges, or parents may provide positive reinforcement and/or response cost based on a "daily report card" the teacher sends home that rates the child's performance that day on selected target behaviors.

■ FAMILY TREATMENT

Role of the Family in Treatment

Attempts to treat disorders in children or adolescents without considering the persons with whom they live or have significant relationships are doomed to failure. Any change in one family member, whether a result of a psychiatric disorder, psychiatric treatment, normal developmental process, or life events, will affect other family members and their relationships. Family constellations vary immensely, from the traditional nuclear family to grandparents functioning as parents, a single-parent family (with or without contact with a second parent), a stepfamily, an adoptive or foster family, or a group home. The term *parents* refers here to adults filling the parenting role regardless of their biological or legal relationship to the patient.

Supportive therapy with families includes counseling in methods of changing behavior; encouraging more positive and realistic parental feelings and attitudes toward children; helping family members to manage their emotional reactions to the child's psychiatric disorder; detecting and obtaining treatment for psychiatric disorders in parents and siblings; and advising parents about schools, treatment modalities, community or leisure activities, and sometimes complex custody and placement decisions.

Family Therapy

Indications

There is consistent empirical support for the effectiveness of family-based interventions for externalizing problems (including adolescent substance abuse), and there is emerging evidence for anxiety and depression as well.

Family therapy may be particularly useful when dysfunctional interactions or impaired communication within the family appear to be related to the presenting problem or when symptoms begin or worsen with a new developmental stage or a change in the family such as divorce, remarriage, adoption, or foster placement. If more than one family member has symptoms, family therapy may be more efficient and effective than multiple individual treatments. It should be considered when one family member improves with treatment but another, not in treatment, worsens. Cases in which the identified patient is relatively unmotivated to participate or to change are likely to be more successful in family therapy than in individual therapy. Attention to family systems issues may be useful when progress is stalled in individual therapy or in behavior therapy. Often family therapy is part of a multimodal treatment plan.

If patients have clearly organic physical or mental illness or if the family equilibrium is precarious and one or more family members are at serious risk for decompensation, family therapy may be useful in combination with other treatments, such as medication or hospitalization. A patient who is acutely psychotic, violent, or delusional regarding the family should not be included in family therapy sessions. Family sessions may not be helpful when a parent has severe but unworkable psychiatric disturbance or when the child or adolescent strongly prefers individual treatment. Children should not be included in family sessions when parents continue (despite redirection) to criticize them or to share inappropriate information, when the most critical issues are marital, or when parents primarily need specific concrete help with practical affairs or parent training. Cultural sensitivity and competence are even more important when working with families than with individuals.

Types of Family Therapy

Structural family therapy.   Structural family therapy (developed by Minuchin) has been the model most used and studied in families in which a child or an adolescent is the identified patient. Its focus is on the present; the identified patient's symptoms are seen as serving a function for the family. The assessment process includes mapping the structure of the family, including the location and permeability of boundaries between family members and around the family and its subsystems. Other important variables are the character and flexibility of alignments of family members, including alliances (joining two or more members in a common interest or task) and coalitions (joint actions directed against one or more family members). Data are gathered on communication patterns and the distribution of power within the family and on the family's sources of stress and support in the environment.

The therapist uses assigned tasks and his or her own interactions with family members to influence the family to change its structure and thereby its functioning, resulting in resolution of the presenting symptoms. Relabeling (i.e., redefining a behavior or symptom to give it a different, usually less negative, meaning for the family) opens alternative pathways for family interactions.

Multigenerational family therapy.   Multigenerational family therapy (pioneered by Murray Bowen) emphasizes how current patterns in families repeat the past. Change results from exploring parents' families of origin and the relationships of the nuclear family to the extended family. Grandparents are often involved indirectly or even brought into the sessions.

Other types.   There are other types of family therapy programs used for specific circumstances such as *family grief therapy, in-home family preservation services, infant or toddler–parent interactive psychotherapy,* and *family approaches for chronic physical illness.* Models that have been used to treat conduct disorders include Patterson's *behavioral family therapy;* Alexander's *functional family therapy,* which combines behavioral and family systems theories and techniques with attention to cognitive processes; and *multisystemic therapy,* developed by Henggeler and Borduin, which uses various home-based therapeutic techniques (family therapy, parent training, and cognitive-behavior therapy) along with direct practical assistance to the family in the context of the adolescent's natural environment of home, school, and neighborhood. For eating disorders, *Maudsley family therapy* is used (see Chapter 5).

Psychoeducational family therapy.   Psychoeducational family therapy, developed for families of adult schizophrenic patients, has been extended to families of patients with childhood disorders, such as eating disorders, ADHD, and anxiety and mood disorders. Detailed didactic presentations about the disorder are designed to enhance the family's support networks and to improve the family's coping skills through increased understanding of the illness, its treatment, and home behavior management techniques. Ongoing treatment uses family systems interventions when educational and behavioral techniques are blocked by dysfunctional family structures or processes. Multiple family group interventions are also used in various treatment programs, including eating disorders, inpatient, or partial hospitalization programs.

■ GROUP THERAPY

Indications

Group therapy may be particularly useful for children and adolescents, who are often more willing to reveal their thoughts and feelings to peers than to adults. Forming rewarding peer relationships is one of the most crucial developmental tasks, which is often difficult for youngsters with psychiatric disorders. Group therapy offers unparalleled opportunities for the clinician to evaluate behavior with peers and for young people to observe and practice important social skills and to benefit from companionship and mutual support. Observations by peers may have a far more acute and powerful effect than those by an adult therapist. Often target symptoms such as aggression, withdrawal, shyness, and/or deficient social skills with peers are not apparent or accessible to intervention in individual therapy. Group therapy may be used as the sole treatment modality, but it is often combined with another treatment. Groups may be helpful as part of the evaluation, particularly for preschool-age children. Structured treatment such as CBT or IPT for depressed adolescents may be efficiently provided in groups.

Group psychotherapy is contraindicated for extremely fragile youngsters and those who are acutely depressed or anxious, psychotic, and/or paranoid. Adolescents with sociopathic traits or behaviors should not be included in groups with others who might be victimized or intimidated. Severely aggressive or hyperactive children should probably not be included in outpatient groups because of the difficulty in controlling their behavior, the risk of their modeling of problem behaviors for other children, and their intimidation of less assertive children.

All of the theoretical models used in individual therapy may be used in group therapy. Therapy may be exclusively verbal or may include expressive arts techniques (such as psychodrama, dance, or arts and crafts), sports activities, or behavioral techniques (such as anger management skills, modeling and practicing social skills, cooperation, and negotiation). Whatever the type of group, the therapist must understand the dynamics of group process. Psychoeducation and supportive treatment can be provided efficiently in groups. Multifamily groups are often used on inpatient units or partial hospitalization programs.

Technical Considerations

Composition

Support groups include members who share a single stressor (e.g., sexual abuse, parental divorce, a chronic physical illness, loss of a loved one). Other groups are specifically targeted to a single psychiatric disorder. Groups that focus on social skills work best with a mixture of patients.

Groups conducted in special schools, inpatient units, or day hospitals are typically open ended and often include all children enrolled in the program, with youth typically grouped by age. Special topic groups focusing on anger management and problem-solving skills, cognitive behavior techniques, substance use, social skills, abuse-related issues, or preparation for discharge from the program also may be offered.

The outpatient group therapist interviews prospective group members individually to assess suitability for the group, to orient the patient to the goals and methods of the group, to learn more about the patient, and to begin to develop a therapeutic alliance between the patient and the leader. Interviewing the parent(s) is also helpful for similar reasons. The younger the child, the more important is parental cooperation.

Group members should be in the same or adjacent developmental stages. Children and adolescents change so dramatically as they develop that an age span broader than 2 or 3 years is unlikely to result in a therapeutic group process. Developmental stage is often more important than chronological age in forming groups for pre- and early adolescents because girls may be more mature than boys in physical and social development related to pubertal onset, and development varies greatly even within the same gender.

Opinions differ on including boys and girls in the same group. Some issues might be better handled in single-sex groups, although children and adolescents may need more focus on getting along with opposite-sex siblings and peers. Combining boys and girls, although initially more difficult, may ultimately be more productive, depending on the setting.

Duration and Goals

Some groups have a defined, limited duration, from 6 weeks to an academic year; others are long term. Short-term groups focus on "current and explicit behavior, adaptation, coping, competency, strengths and growth…. [With] emphasis on the dynamics of the here-and-now corrective emotional experience, [and] on the patients' active participation in the change effort" (Scheidlinger 1984, p. 581). Long-term groups are more likely to aim for the promotion of insight, the resolution of unconscious conflicts, and the removal of developmental arrests.

Leadership

Of all modalities of therapy, the need for co-therapists is most clear in group treatment. Groups are complex, with many events occurring simultaneously, and a second observer is valuable. In groups of younger children, an extra pair of hands is needed. Co-leaders who differ from each other in age, sex, race, or culture may expand the opportunities for different types of patient–therapist relationships.

Rules

The group structure should fit the nature of the group and the patients. A psychodynamically oriented discussion group for depressed or anxious adolescents will need far fewer rules than a group that aims to teach social skills to school-age boys with conduct problems. The leaders are responsible for maintaining structure and control of behavior within the group. At times, strategies such as the time-out may even be required. The leaders must be explicit about the rules of confidentiality for the group because the group setting increases the risk of breach of confidentiality.

Family Contact

Involving parents is especially important for preschool- and school-age children in order to identify important events in the child's environment and to monitor progress. Adolescents are more willing and able to report and are also more sensitive to confidentiality issues. For children of all ages, the therapist should inform parents of the general goals of the group and their child's progress toward specific goals. Parent education in development and behavior management is often provided most efficiently in a coordinated parent group session. Parents may also appreciate the opportunity to meet with other parents whose children have similar problems.

Developmental Issues

Groups for Preschool-Age Children

Young children are less able to verbalize and require more structure and planned activities than older children. A group can provide a powerful context to teach social skills and language, especially for children who have pervasive developmental disorder or developmental delays.

Groups for School-Age Children

Because school-age children have great difficulty bringing in outside material for discussion or engaging in introspection, verbal portions of the group can focus on events that occur in the group itself. Games and craft activities can provide a useful structure, but the leader(s) must ensure that recreation does not become the only function of the group. Behavior modification, cognitive problem-solving techniques, and anger management skills may be efficacious. Many child patients will not spontaneously attempt to relate to other children. Others have been rejected or scapegoated by peers. If the group is successful, the children will be able to generalize the skills learned to form relationships with peers at school and in their neighborhoods.

Children with ADHD are often referred to group therapy because of their difficulty with peer relationships and their lack of insight into their difficulties. Children who are taking stimulant medication may need to receive a dose before the group meets to help them benefit from the group therapy and not disrupt it for others.

Groups for Adolescents

Cognitive-behavioral group treatment (CBT) for adolescents and parents has been shown to be an effective treatment of depression (Brent et al. 1997; Lewinsohn et al. 1990). Such groups have been adapted for teens with anxiety disorders as well. Similar groups may help prevent depression in teenagers at risk. Twelve-step groups are used for adolescents who have problems with drug or alcohol abuse. DBT includes a group format.

Many adolescent groups can be conducted as exclusively verbal discussion groups, although some activities may help to break the ice. If both boys and girls are included in the same group, the leaders should attempt to equalize the gender ratio as much as possible and be alert to sexual undercurrents and acting out, while facilitating the discussion of sexual concerns and the practicing of social skills.

■ WRAPAROUND SERVICES

Innovative community services, often called "wraparound" programs, are used to avoid hospitalization or placement in residential treatment. Such services attempt to address complex needs (psychological, school, family, peer, spiritual) in a strength-based community model. Wraparound services involve a variety of interventions with individualized programming and therapy, active involvement of family and community members, integration with social services (such as child welfare, financial support, and housing), and use of interventions in the home, neighborhood, community, and school rather than in the traditional office or hospital setting. Crisis intervention teams, brief respite placement, and in-home therapy/supervision are typically included. Funding sources vary depending on the specific community or state.

■ HOSPITALIZATION AND RESIDENTIAL TREATMENT

Indications

Because children and adolescents should be treated in the setting that is least restrictive and disruptive to their lives, hospital or residential treatment is reserved for youngsters who have not responded to outpatient treatment because of severity of symptoms, lack of motivation, outright resistance, or severe disorganization of the patient or family. If there is concomitant physical illness requiring skilled medical/nursing care, hospitalization may also be necessary. In cases where seeking of psychiatric services has been delayed, more complex and severe symptoms may demand more intensive treatment from the onset, even before outpatient services are attempted.

Hospitalization is usually an acute event that is precipitated by immediate physical danger to self or others, acute psychosis, a crisis in the environment that reduces the ability of the caregiving adults to cope with the child or adolescent, or failure of less intensive forms of treatment. Some hospitalizations are needed for a more intensive, systematic, and detailed evaluation and observation of the patient and family than is possible in an outpatient or a day treatment program or if the patient is resistant to outpatient or day treatment. Over the past decades, hospital lengths of stay have become much shorter. With exceptions only for the most severely ill youngsters, hospitalization is now typically used only to stabilize the acute clinical situation and to arrange for treatment in a less restrictive setting. Placement in a residential treatment center may be indicated for children and adolescents with chronic behavior problems such as aggression, running away, truancy, substance abuse, school refusal, or self-destructive acts that the family, foster home, and/or community cannot manage.

Components of Treatment

Pharmacotherapy

Hospitalization offers an ideal opportunity for systematic trials of medications in children or adolescents whose conditions have not responded to conventional treatment, who have complicated or unclear diagnoses, who have medical problems complicating pharmacotherapy, or whose parents are not able to reliably administer medication and report on efficacy and side effects.

Individual Psychotherapy

As newer treatment methods have evolved and hospital stays have become shorter, individual psychotherapy is less often used as an inpatient primary treatment modality. Regularly scheduled individual sessions with a therapist with whom the child or adolescent can develop a trusting relationship continue to be important in developing a more complete understanding of the patient's intrapsychic, familial, and social dynamics and assisting him or her in developing more adaptive methods of coping with strong emotions. The therapist may be able to help the patient address past traumas and losses, better understand his or her own difficulties, and make use of the other treatments offered.

Milieu Therapy

Milieu therapy includes the total environment, in the context of a structured schedule for daily life. It presents a valuable opportunity to observe the patient over an extended period during meals, sleep, self-care, and play. Goals of the milieu include using clear rules and a regular routine to promote a sense of security and predictability and teaching of specific skills to increase self-esteem and competence. Many settings include a behavioral program that uses a token economy or privilege level system to manage behavior and to modify specific symptoms.

Group Therapy

In addition to general or special topic groups, many programs include community meetings in which therapists set privileges and rules, patients practice social skills, and patients learn to observe their own and others' behavior and to recognize the effect of their behavior on others.

Education

Virtually all children and adolescents who require out-of-home placement have had problems in school. The small classes and highly trained teachers of a hospital unit or residential center school can provide a detailed evaluation of a youngster's academic strengths and weaknesses. One of the most important parts of discharge planning is arranging for an appropriate educational placement and working with the teacher to set appropriate target goals. Youngsters in residential treatment centers are gradually integrated into a special education or mainstream program in the local public or private schools, although some larger residential centers have self-contained classrooms within their facility.

Family Treatment

Work with families is an essential part of hospital treatment. Interventions may include family therapy, parent counseling in behavior management, and education about the nature of the child's disorder and treatment plan. Parents may require marital therapy; individual assessment and treatment; or help with housing, finances, day care, or medical care.

■ DAY TREATMENT

A day hospital or day treatment program, often called partial hospitalization, may be best for children or adolescents who require more intensive intervention than can be provided in outpatient visits but who are able to live at home, in foster care, or in a group home. Compared with hospitalization or residential placement, day treatment is less disruptive to the patient and the family and can offer an opportunity for intensive work with parents, who typically attend the program on a regular basis. Daily planning and review of home management strategies enhance generalization and maintenance of gains made in treatment. A day program may be used to avoid the necessity of inpatient hospitalization, to aggressively address school refusal problems, or as a transition for a patient who has been hospitalized.

Day treatment programs vary in the design, the treatment techniques, and the patient populations, although all treat moderately to severely ill children and adolescents. Some programs provide a full 8-hour day, 5 days a week, and include a school program. When the patients are younger than 6 years, the program may be called a *therapeutic nursery*. Other programs may meet in the late afternoon and evening hours (typically for 3 hours), after patients attend community schools, and on weekends, which facilitates parental attendance. Some agencies offer intensive summer day treatment programs or a therapeutic day camp. The modalities of treatment are variable but tend to be similar to those described for inpatient units; however, the staff-to-patient ratio is often lower. Lengths of stay are decreasing in many day treatment programs, as in inpatient hospitalization.

■ ADJUNCTIVE TREATMENTS

At times, an intervention that is not, strictly speaking, a psychiatric treatment may be recommended as part of a treatment plan. These could include spiritual, recreational, or extracurricular activities. These programs may be crucial to the child's or adolescent's well-being and the treatment of the psychiatric disorder, or they may encourage progress or improve level of functioning.

Special Education Placements

Modified school programs are indicated for children and adolescents who cannot perform satisfactorily in regular classrooms or who need special structure or teaching techniques to reach their academic potential. These programs range in intensity from tutoring or resource classrooms several hours a week, to special classrooms in mainstream schools, to public or private schools that serve only children and adolescents with special educational needs. Resources differ from community to community, but most have programs for mentally retarded youth, for those with learning disabilities (specific developmental disorders), and for those whose emotional and/or behavior problems require a special setting for learning. Classes are small, with a high teacher-to-student ratio and specially trained teachers. Vocational evaluation and education may be crucial, especially for adolescents.

Child and adolescent psychiatrists are being added to the interdisciplinary team as consultants or in school-based health and mental health clinics. These programs efficiently provide coordinated medical and mental health care, although funding can be difficult to maintain.

A boarding school may be useful when a parent–child problem is unresponsive to treatment or an appropriate placement is not available in the home community. Some boarding schools have special programs for children with learning disabilities or psychiatric disorders.

Recreation

Learning to perform a sport or skill competently may be an especially important adjunct to treatment in children and adolescents who lack positive relationships with peers or adults because of social isolation, withdrawal, or being ignored or actively rejected. Trained recreation therapists work in various psychiatric and community settings and focus on teaching adaptive leisure skills and improving interactions with peers. A relationship with an adult such as a Big Brother or Sister or a YMCA counselor or sports coach offers an opportunity to interact with a peer group under supervision and may provide support and build self-esteem until the child or adolescent improves enough to establish relationships independently. Some families have employed a high school or college student one or more afternoons a week to teach the child social and play skills, develop a relationship with the child, and provide structured time. This method also gives parents a respite and an opportunity to spend time with their other children.

Day or overnight summer camps are potentially a very helpful experience. Some youngsters can attend regular camp, whereas others need a therapeutic camp program geared toward children and adolescents with psychiatric or medical problems.

Foster Care

Placement in a foster home may be needed when parents are unwilling or unable to care for their child. Indications are clearest in cases of physical or medical neglect or physical or sexual abuse. Some families may not be able to provide the appropriate emotional nurturance and supervision. Court intervention is required for placement. Foster care should be short term, until parents are rehabilitated or the courts decide that more permanent placement is needed. Unfortunately, child welfare agencies in many communities are overwhelmed, and children and adolescents may require advocacy with the appointment of a *guardian ad litem* attorney to facilitate return to parents, placement in a foster home or group home, or termination of parental rights to free the child for adoption, according to the conditions of the child and family.

Children with severe behavior or physical problems or older adolescents who are difficult to place or maintain in foster or adoptive homes may be placed in group homes with trained staff. These programs vary in staffing and intensity of the treatment offered. Some resemble residential treatment, whereas others simply provide a supervised residence.

Parent Support Groups

Various groups that provide education and support for parents, as well as conduct fund-raising and advocacy for services, have been organized by parents with professional support. Examples are listed in the Appendix. Numerous local groups (many of which are affiliated with national organizations) focus on specific medical or psychiatric disorders or on more generic psychological problems of childhood. They provide a powerful adjunct to more traditional professional services.

■ REFERENCES

Brent DA, Holder D, Kolko D, et al: A clinical psychotherapy trial for adolescent depression comparing cognitive, family, and supportive therapy. Arch Gen Psychiatry 54:877–885, 1997

Gunlicks-Stoessel ML, Mufson L: Interpersonal psychotherapy for depressed adolescents, in Dulcan's Textbook of Child and Adolescent Psychiatry. Edited by Dulcan MK. Washington, DC, American Psychiatric Publishing, 2010, pp 825–844

Kazdin AE: Parent management training: evidence, outcomes, and issues. J Am Acad Child Adolesc Psychiatry 36:1349–1356, 1997

Lewinsohn PM, Clarke GN, Hops H, et al: Cognitive-behavioral treatment for depressed adolescents. Behavior Therapy 21:385–401, 1990

Pelham WE, Murphy HA: Attention deficit and conduct disorders, in Pharmacological and Behavioral Treatment: An Integrative Approach. Edited by Herson M. New York, Wiley, 1986, pp 108–148

Scheidlinger S: Short-term group psychotherapy for children: an overview. Int J Group Psychother 34:573–585, 1984

Strupp HH: Psychotherapy: Clinical Research, and Theoretical Issues. New York, Jason Aronson, 1973

■ ADDITIONAL READING

Barkley RA: Defiant Children: A Clinician's Manual for Assessment and Parent Training, 2nd Edition. New York, Guilford, 1997

Barkley RA, Edwards GH, Robin AL: Defiant Teens: A Clinician's Manual for Assessment and Family Intervention. New York, Guilford, 1999

Chorpita BF: Modular Cognitive-Behavioral Therapy for Childhood Anxiety Disorders. New York, Guilford, 2007

Cohen JA, Mannarino AP, Deblinger E: Treating Trauma and Traumatic Grief in Children and Adolescents. New York, Guilford, 2006

Forehand R, McMahon RJ: Helping the Non-Compliant Child: Family Based Treatment for Oppositional Behavior, 2nd Edition. New York, Guilford, 2003

Greene RW, Ablon JS: Treating Explosive Kids: The Collaborative Problem-Solving Approach. New York, Guilford, 2006

Henggeler SW, Schoenwald SK, Borduin CM, et al: Multisystemic Therapy for Antisocial Behavior in Children and Adolescents, 2nd Edition. New York, Guilford, 2009

Mendenhall AN, Arnold LE, Fristad MA: Parent counseling, psychoeducation, and parent support groups, in Dulcan's Textbook of Child and Adolescent Psychiatry. Edited by Dulcan MK.Washington, DC, American Psychiatric Publishing, 2010, pp 825–844

Miller AL, Rathus HK, Linehan MM: Dialectical Behavior Therapy With Suicidal Adolescents. New York, Guilford, 2007

Mufson L, Dorta KP, Moreau D, et al: Interpersonal Psychotherapy for Depressed Adolescents, 2nd Edition. New York, Guilford, 2004

Nagy P: Motivational interviewing, in Dulcan's Textbook of Child and Adolescent Psychiatry. Edited by Dulcan MK. Washington, DC, American Psychiatric Publishing, 2010, pp 915–924

Petti TA: Milieu treatment: inpatient, partial hospitalization, and residential programs, in Dulcan's Textbook of Child and Adolescent Psychiatry. Edited by Dulcan MK. Washington, DC, American Psychiatric Publishing, 2010, pp 939–953

Reinecke MA, Dattilio FM, Freeman A (eds): Cognitive Therapy With Children and Adolescents: A Casebook for Clinical Practice, 2nd Edition. New York, Guilford, 2003

Strayhorn JM: The Competent Child: An Approach to Psychotherapy and Preventive Mental Health. New York, Guilford, 1988

Terr L: Magical Moments of Change: How Psychotherapy Turns Kids Around. New York, WW Norton, 2008

Webster-Stratton C, Herbert M: Troubled Families–Problem Children. New York, Wiley, 1994

Wendel R, Gouze KR: Family therapy. Dulcan's Textbook of Child and Adolescent Psychiatry. Edited by Dulcan MK. Washington, DC, American Psychiatric Publishing, 2010, pp 869–886

Appendix

RESOURCES FOR PARENTS

■ INFORMATION ON THE INTERNET

American Academy of Child and Adolescent Psychiatry
3615 Wisconsin Ave., N.W.
Washington, D.C. 20016
http://www.aacap.org

- *Facts for Families—information sheets written for the general public on development, problem behaviors, stressors, and psychiatric disorders. Available also in Spanish and Polish.*
- *Resource Centers*
- *Guides for parents*

Autism Society of America
4340 East-West Highway, Suite 350
Bethesda, MD 20814
800-3-AUTISM
http://www.autism-society.org

Bright Futures
http://www.brightfutures.org
Publications to promote and improve the health and well-being of children and adolescents.

Note. As scientific research advances, information and advice change. Many topics are controversial, even among experts. Parents should be encouraged to discuss questions with their child's pediatrician, child and adolescent psychiatrist, or other health or mental health professional.

Child and Adolescent Bipolar Foundation
http://www.bpkids.org

Child Mind Institute
http://www.childmind.org

Children and Adults With Attention-Deficit/Hyperactivity Disorder (CHADD)
8181 Professional Place, Suite 150
Landover, MD 20785
301-306-7070
http://www.chadd.org
Includes National Resource Center on AD/HD

Learning Disabilities Association of America
http://www.ldanatl.org

National Alliance on Mental Illness (NAMI)
3803 N. Fairfax Drive, Suite 100
Arlington, VA 22203
703-524-7600
http://www.nami.org

National Federation of Families for Children's Mental Health
9605 Medical Center Drive
Rockville, MD 20850
240-403-1901
http://www.ffcmh.org

National Institute of Mental Health
http://www.nimh.nih.gov

Online Asperger Syndrome Information and Support (OASIS)
http://www.aspergersyndrome.org

Tourette Syndrome Association
42-40 Bell Boulevard
Bayside, NY 11361
1-718-224-2999
http://www.tsa-usa.org

Zero to Three
Developmental information for parents of children ages 4 years and younger, including how to enhance children's learning and social–emotional growth.
http://www.zerotothree.org

■ BOOKS

Child Development

American Academy of Child and Adolescent Psychiatry: Your Child: What Every Parent Needs to Know. New York, Harper Collins, 1998
American Academy of Child and Adolescent Psychiatry: Your Adolescent: Emotional, Behavioral and Cognitive Development From Early Adolescence Through the Teen Years. New York, Harper Collins, 1999

Managing Child Behavior

Barkley RA, Benton CM: Your Defiant Child: 8 Steps to Better Behavior. New York, Guilford, 1998
Barkley RA, Robin AL: Your Defiant Teen: 10 Steps to Resolve Conflict and Rebuild Your Relationship. New York, Guilford, 2008
Clark L: SOS! Help for Parents: A Practical Guide for Handling Common Everyday Behavior Problems, 2nd Edition. Bowling Green, KY, Parents Press, 1985
Faber A, Mazlish E: How to Talk So Kids Will Listen and Listen So Kids Will Talk. New York, HarperCollins, 1980
Forehand R, Long N: Parenting the Strong-Willed Child: The Clinically Proven Five-Week Program for Parents of Two- to Six-Year-Olds, 3rd Edition. New York, McGraw-Hill, 2010
Ginott HG: Between Parent and Child. Revised and updated by Ginott A, Goddard HW. New York, Three Rivers Press, 2003

Green RW: The Explosive Child: A New Approach for Understanding and Parenting Easily Frustrated, Chronically Inflexible Children. New York, HarperCollins, 2010

Kazdin AE: The Kazdin Method for Parenting the Defiant Child. New York, Mariner Books, 2009 (includes a DVD)

Phelan TW: 1–2–3 Magic: Effective Discipline for Children 2–12, 3rd Edition. Glen Ellyn, IL, ParentMagic, 2003

Anger Management for Parents

Clark L: SOS! Help for Emotions: Managing Anxiety, Anger, and Depression, 2nd Edition. Bowling Green, KY, Parents Press, 2002

Psychiatric Disorders

Anxiety

Foa EB, Andrews LW: If Your Adolescent Has an Anxiety Disorder: An Essential Resource for Parents. New York, Oxford University Press, 2006

Manassis K: Keys to Parenting Your Anxious Child. Hauppauge, NY, Barron's Educational Series, 1996

March JS: Talking Back to OCD. New York, Guilford, 2007

McHolm AE, Cunningham CE, Vanier MK: Helping Your Child with Selective Mutism: Practical Steps to Overcome a Fear of Speaking. Oakland, CA, New Harbinger Publications, 2005

Rapee RM, Spence SH, Cobham V, et al: Helping Your Anxious Child: A Step-by-Step Guide for Parents. Oakland, CA, New Harbinger Publications, 2000

Attention-Deficit/Hyperactivity Disorder

American Academy of Pediatrics: ADHD: A Complete and Authoritative Guide. Elk Grove Village, IL, American Academy of Pediatrics, 2004

Barkley R: Taking Charge of ADHD: The Complete, Authoritative Guide for Parents, Revised Edition. New York, Guilford, 2000

Jensen PS: Making the System Work for Your Child With ADHD. New York, Guilford, 2004

Zeigler Dendy, CA: Teenagers with ADD and ADHD: A Guide for Parents and Professionals, 2nd Edition. Bethesda, MD, Woodbine House, 2006

Autism and Asperger's Disorder

Attwood T: The Complete Guide to Asperger's Syndrome. Philadelphia, PA, Jessica Kingsley Publishers, 2007

Siegel B: Getting the Best for Your Child With Autism: An Expert's Guide to Treatment. New York, Guilford, 2008

Depression and Bipolar Disorder

Birmaher B: New Hope for Children and Teens With Bipolar Disorder. New York, Three Rivers Press, 2004

Evans DL, Andrews LW: If Your Adolescent Has Depression or Bipolar Disorder: An Essential Resource for Parents. New York, Oxford University Press, 2005

Fristad MA, Arnold JSG: Raising a Moody Child: How to Cope With Depression and Bipolar Disorder. New York, Guilford, 2004

Miklowitz DJ, George EL: The Bipolar Teen: What You Can Do to Help Your Child and Your Family. New York, Guilford, 2008

Eating Disorders

Lock J, Le Grange, D: Help Your Teenager Beat an Eating Disorder. New York, Guilford, 2005

Walsh BT, Cameron VL: If Your Adolescent Has an Eating Disorder: An Essential Resource for Parents. New York, Oxford University Press, 2005

Tourette's Disorder

Parker JN, Parker PM (eds): The Official Parent's Sourcebook on Tourette Syndrome: A Revised and Updated Directory for the Internet Age. San Diego, CA, ICON Health Publications, 2002

Psychiatric Medication

Dulcan MK (ed): Helping Parents, Youth, and Teachers Understand Medications for Behavioral and Emotional Problems: A Resource Book of Medication Information Handouts, 3rd Edition. Washington, DC, American Psychiatric Publishing, 2007

Wilens TE: Straight Talk About Psychiatric Medications for Kids, 3rd Edition. New York, Guilford, 2009

INDEX

*Page numbers printed in **boldface** type refer to tables or figures.*

352